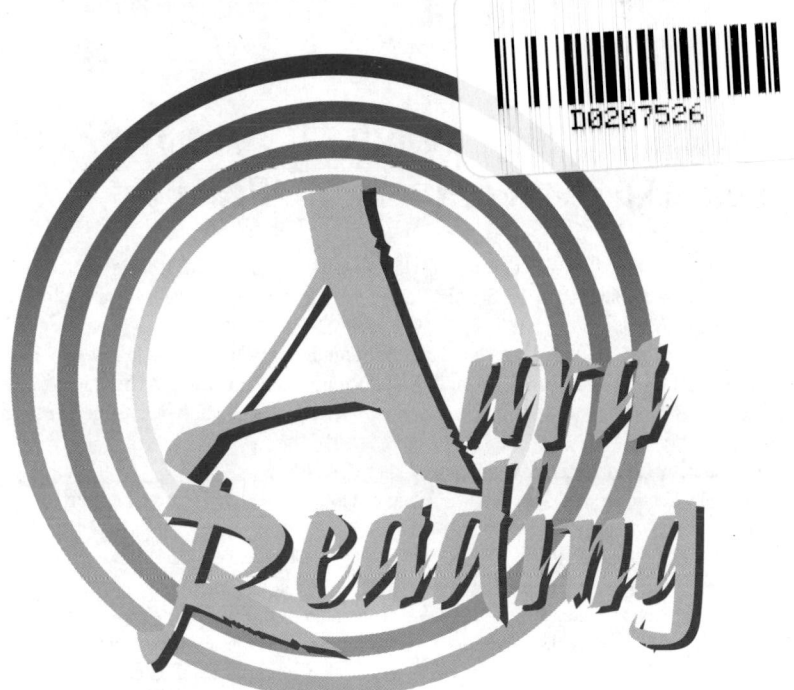

Aura Reading

Through ALL Your Senses

Celestial Perception Made Practical

Rose Rosetree

WOMEN'S INTUITION WORLDWIDE
www.rose-rosetree.com

Aura Reading Through All Your Senses: Celestial Perception Made Practical

Publisher's Cataloging-in-Publication
(Provided by Quality Books, Inc.)

    Rosetree, Rose.
        Aura reading through all your senses / Rose Rosetree.
    -- 2nd ed.
        p. cm.
        Includes bibliographical references and index.
        ISBN-13: 978-0-9651145-4-7
        ISBN-10: 0-9651145-4-6
        1. Aura. 2. Chakras. 3. Intuition (Psychology)
    I. Title.
    BF1389.A8R6 2004   133.8'92
                           QBI01-201007

Website and blog at www.rose-rosetree.com
Inquiries for quantity discounts, foreign rights sales,
personal sessions, media interviews, and workshops:
rights@rose-rosetree.com or 703-404-4357

To those who are skeptical but curious,
To those who are curious but intimidated,
To those who are brilliant aura readers
but don't know it yet.

Foreword

This book invites you to upgrade your skill at reading auras, whether you're a newbie or an experienced aura reader with the desire to keep growing.

Since this how-to was published eight years ago, people keep having better results with the method of Aura Reading Through All Your Senses. I believe it's because our human family is evolving extra fast now so that we can fulfill a prophesy given by wisdom traditions from many parts of the world.

A thousand years of enlightenment and peace have been predicted to begin by the year 2012. If I could choose (and maybe I have), I'd prefer being part of the transition team... not just living a glorious life but able to appreciate it deeply, having known the full meaning of human fear and pain.

Whether or not an Age of Enlightenment eventually dawns, there's no question that reading auras before then takes courage. I began with secret fears of being the one student who couldn't learn. Worse, I dreaded that my aura itself would look so pathetic that my teacher, reading every student in turn, would mumble to me something like, "Sorry about that."

Since then, I've learned that every human aura reveals exquisite, distinctive gifts of the soul. So not to worry. Even if one of your chakras shows that, along with a gift, you have room for growth, what's so horrible about that? Finding a problem is better than denying it; moreover, any blockage in auras can always be released, and sometimes all it takes is one good prayer. Here's the bottom line: Your aura is magnificent.

So don't be shy about using the glorious gifts inscribed there. For every hundred people today who are skeptics, for every dozen people who'd rather give their power away to a so-called "expert" on spiritual matters than read the truth for themselves, there's one courageous person like you—someone willing to risk the insecurity of learning—a rising aura reader.

For 33 years now, I've served as a spiritual teacher. If the pattern I've seen holds true, students (including me, not just you) will remain students. But we'll also be invited to teach. Hundreds, maybe thousands, of people will be coming to *you* in the next decade. And they won't be fooling around. They'll have a very real need to learn what you can tell them. Get ready.

Rose Rosetree
Sterling, Virginia, July 2004

Contents

Table of Techniques

Development of your celestial perception can move you into a higher state of consciousness in everyday life. So this book is loaded with techniques to wake up your celestial perception. All listings are for the first page where a technique is explained.

Some of the techniques that follow will be described at length and referred to repeatedly (for additional references, see the index). Other techniques will be mentioned only briefly. But don't overlook their apparent simplicity. If you feel invited to try them, your curiosity will be amply rewarded. Use this table to locate all topics of special interest to you.

Chapter 1

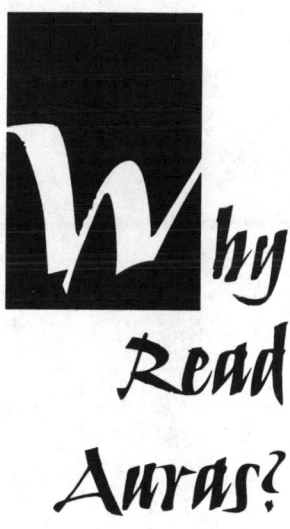

Why Read Auras?

*H*ow would your life change if you could read auras? In ways big and small, you would gain knowledge of spiritual truth. That much perhaps you already know. But do you also appreciate that aura reading can bring you down-to-earth benefits? Ordinary things turn amazing, from kissing babies to playing with puppies. If you thought your TV was in color before, wait until you turn on the auras.

Yes, auras can be watched on TV. Photos in your daily newspaper, snapshots of family reunions, your favorite baby picture that shows you with chocolate pudding smeared all over your face—all of these have auras. And you can definitely learn to read them.

So people have auras, not only in person but when their images are captured on film. Could plants have auras too?

Only the live ones. Here's where aura reading begins to turn into knowledge that brings you consumer bonus points.

Who hasn't had this experience? You splurge on a bouquet of long-stemmed red roses. In the store they look gorgeous. But, once you bring them home, the poor things never open their buds. Displaying a total lack of romance, your roses shrivel up and die.

How could they?

Energetically, the flowers were half dead when you bought them. Had you read their auras, you would have known.

Gardeners really appreciate the information from auras, both for choosing healthy plants and for keeping them alive. You'll read more about this later.

One kind of plant is especially important to read, the edible kind. Any food, vegetable or animal, contains life energy. Or should! This book gives you many techniques for exploring the life in food.

Bitter eggplants; grapefruits with an unpleasantly sour taste; oranges that are part juicy, part shrivelled—when you buy this stuff don't you feel like a sucker? As an aura reader, you can know better. One application of aura reading is to taste food without physically biting into it.

Mindblowing, huh? But my students have learned to do all this and more. You can too. I think you'll especially enjoy another one of my discoveries about aura reading: smelling perfume through more than one sense. And without opening the bottle. A later chapter will show you how.

Any products for personal use affect your personal aura. Therefore, you can apply techniques of aura reading to test whether or not specific products will work well on you. Test before you buy.

Shampoo, deodorant, hand lotion—no manufactured product can guarantee the same results for everyone. Chemistry happens. With toiletries I figure it's like the disclaimer for cars: Your actual mileage may vary.

So don't be embarrassed at all those times you've bought toiletries that turned out to be unreturnable duds. (Do you throw these mistakes straight into the garbage or do what I used to do—pile them into a closet for several years and then throw them out?) Aura reading can cut down on these frustrating wastes of money.

Consuming means two things: shopping *and* enjoying. After you've used aura reading to fill your shopping cart wisely, the best is yet to come. Enjoyment of your purchases grows when you explore how they change your aura.

For instance, later in this book you'll find techniques to explore what music does to your energy field. And there's an entire chapter devoted to aura reading as a means to better health.

Secrets About People in Your Life

What an understatement to call aura reading fun! As if it weren't fascinating enough to plunge into the auric effects of the Beatles, Chanel No. 5, and your favorite flavor of ice cream, imagine what happens when you can read auras of your family and friends. Auras reveal juicy stuff about what is really going on with people in areas like love and communication.

Auras can tell you more, in the here and now, than any other system you have used thus far to gain insight into people.

- Wish you could screen dates better? Gather a month's worth of insights from one 15-minute aura reading.

- Stuck in a rut with neighbors, relatives, even your best friend? Discover new dimensions when you read their fascinating energy fields.

- People at work starting to drive you nuts? Aura reading might be able to help there, too.

You get the idea. If you're a people person, you've been waiting for this kind of knowledge all your life.

Today trust is a major motivator for people to observe others more closely. So aura reading is a timely discovery. You see, auras always tell the truth. In fact, this book contains some very specific lie detector tests.

Auras contain so much truth, in fact, that reading them offers significant advantages for all your relationships, no matter how intimate. Share with your mate the techniques for applying aura reading to sex, massage, and more.

Auras become a matter of passionate interest when you realize how much there is to them. They show levels within people that go far beyond what you expect, even what you could imagine. Psychology, philosophy, even religion may not have prepared you for the immediate experience of truth that auras can bring you.

Celestial perception is one name for this. Celestial—that means the realm of angels, of deep human secrets. Aura reading can move you into this higher state of consciousness where, at will, you can enter into an experience of soul-stirring beauty. Did you know that a tender, exquisite presence can be found in any human aura? Mystics have called it Divine.

What language do you use now to describe what makes people unique at their deepest level? Perhaps you use words like these: Individuality. Soul. Suchness. Essence. Otherness. Whatever you call it, aura reading leads you to experience That in all its humbling glory.

Can You Really Do It?

"But can I really do it?" So many students have asked me this outright. Even more have worried silently. Well, not to worry. Do you have the desire to read auras? Do you own this book? It offers you more than a hundred techniques and tips. Will you give them a chance, one a day, as if you were taking vitamins? If so, you've got all it takes to become an aura reader.

In *The Celestine Prophecy*, James Redfield writes about the importance of becoming more spiritually aware. He calls it *"engaging the energy"* and goes on to suggest that the more actively we engage this spiritual energy, the happier we'll feel. Meaningful coincidence will increase. And our personal evolution will help humanity reach the critical mass that is needed to bring about Heaven on Earth.

Becoming an aura reader is the obvious next step for the millions of Americans who were inspired by Redfield's vision. Development of your subtle perception can lift you into a higher state of consciousness.

But as good a beginning as Redfield presented, his novel was never designed to offer a complete, systematic how-to on aura reading. In recent years, many students who have come to this teacher's classes were frustrated because they loved *The Celestine Prophecy* but wanted to experience auras, not just read about them. Without exception, the method of Aura Reading Through All Your Senses has brought them to clear perception.

Reading auras requires two things really, perception and interpretation. Both are easy with this book's techniques because the approach involves letting go. Commonly, students are taught to force and strain instead. This seldom works.

Discover Talents You Never Knew You Had

Another innovative aspect of *Aura Reading Through All Your Senses* is a form of self-discovery that can greatly accelerate your progress as an aura reader. **This is the first book to identify 11 different subtle senses that can be used for aura reading.**

Other approaches to auras focus primarily on clairvoyance, the gift of subtle sight. That's useful but other subtle senses can serve you just as well.

Could you be an empath without even knowing it? Learning to handle this gift could mean a life-changing breakthrough for you, as it has for many of my clients. Natural empaths often suffer a great deal until they learn how to become *skilled* empaths. Information given in the next chapter could make all the difference in the world. (To perform a significant act of friendship, give this book to anyone you suspect may be an empath.)

Intense emotional sensitivity isn't the only gift that makes for superb aura reading. Equally important gifts can show as an apparent lack of sensitivity. Truth knowledge, for instance, may cause a person to come across like an absent-minded professor. That individual may not appear especially sensuous (except in the midst of a great meal or a hot date—after all, we all have our moments). Ironically, people who don't seem especially in touch with the down-to-earth stuff could be highly talented at *subtle* sensing.

When you read descriptions of all 11 potential gifts for aura reading, you may receive one of the major surprises of your life.

Something you may have dismissed as a personal quirk, something you have taken for granted, something you never thought was important could bring you outstanding results as an aura reader.

Identifying yourself as having even 1 of these 11 spiritual gifts could transform your self-esteem and align other aspects of your personality. In ways that transcend aura reading, you could birth a new you.

And it's a sure bet that knowledge about subtle gifts has been lacking in your prior education. You could be a prominent psychiatrist, a professional negotiator, or the world's champion surfer on the Internet yet still not have a clue about some of your most intimate intuitive talents. Learning about them could change your sense of identity forever.

Remember the story of "The Ugly Duckling"? He turned out not to be ugly at all ... once he realized that he actually was a swan. Things that bother *you* in everyday life may be tipoffs to special sensitivity related to your spiritual gifts. Thus, the very problems that weigh you down could be related to your highest inspiration.

The trick is to understand what on earth these spiritual gifts are, then identify and use them.

- Michael describes himself as a touchy-feely person. He has developed this label in self-defense to cover a certain amount of embarrassment. Truth is, Michael doesn't feel complete unless he shakes people's hands, shares some human contact. And when people don't consider this proper, which is fairly often, Michael holds back. Then he feels frustrated, even guilty.

Surprise! Michael has an exceptionally strong gift for *clairsentience*, subtle touch.

- Beth hates making decisions. She tortures herself by seeing "too many" possibilities. So Beth works hard at squelching the impulse to see things from more than one side. Ironically even when she succeeds, it feels like failure.

Surprise! Beth's *analytical awareness* is a wonderful asset for aura reading. And when she learns to use her gift in this way, for once she can use it fully. This brings a profound sense of relief.

- Dozens of times each day, Alexander wants to butt in. Much as he hates to annoy people at work, at the gym, wherever he goes, annoyance grows until he just has to say something. "Please turn that music down." "Does the TV have to be so loud?"

Evidently other people are better at tuning out background noise. No matter how hard he tries, it drives him crazy. Secretly Alexander worries. Maybe this thing about him and noise really *is* crazy.

Surprise! There's nothing crazy at all about *clairaudience*, the gift of subtle hearing. Aura reading gives Alexander a situation where he can take his gift as far as it can go.

You see, subtle senses demand to be used. Unrecognized talent is more than a waste. It pesters us in stupid little ways until we acknowledge the talent and put it to positive use.

Find Your Way In

The bottom line is for you to be able to find your personal *way in* to subtle perception.

Everyone has this *way in*—a knack, like a button that only you can push to open the door to a secret passageway. Finding this knack may seem like magic. But in retrospect you'll discover that it has involved three simple steps: You need to identify your gifts for subtle sensing, direct them in an appropriate manner, and let go.

> **After you find your way in,
> there will be no stopping you.**

Over the past ten years, I've seen this happen to my students. Some have never tried aura reading before. Most have tried and failed. A few have seen some colors but weren't sure what they meant. Repeatedly, the method of Aura Reading Through All Your Senses has shown that **everyone can learn to read auras**.

So what holds people back? The widespread *myth about auras* confuses most people who have heard it and, usually, leads to a state of chronic psychic shutdown.

When you read the next chapter, you'll find out how much of this myth has crept into your own mind. The next chapter also helps you clear away the myth, replacing it with a truth that can serve you better.

Beginner's techniques will guide you, then, to find your way in. Aha! the light of understanding can go on for good. Based on this, a sequence of increasingly sophisticated techniques will help you discover more and more.

You'll come to realize that **aura reading is more than the watered-down use of intuition that most folks settle for in everyday life.** "I have a feeling" is okay, but don't let that be as far as you take your priceless gifts for subtle perception. Similarly some folks learn to see a layer or two of aura around people. It's there all the time and that's nice, but so what? This hardly amounts to an aura reading; it's just a good start.

As you'll discover from using the systematic sequence of techniques from Chapter Three onward, aura reading can clue you in to highly specific insights that you can use ... like Superman.

Superman—remember how he could see through things? Sure, he could also fly and bend steel bars as though they were wads of bubble gum. Seeing auras won't help you do that. On the other hand, with the kind of superpowers we'll awaken together, you'll be able to see through—or into—nearly anything. And without risking a headache from kryptonite.

Aura Reading Through All Your Senses **can restore a wholeness to life that, though not superhuman, is more than most adults today know as human life.**

When you use celestial perception on a daily basis, when you can turn it on or off at will as with the flick of a light switch, then you can evaluate the significance of the truth now available to you. Are auras heavenly or human or both? For that matter, which is your life?

Expectations of Flash

Unrealistic expectations of flashy experience sometimes get in the way for beginning aura readers. TV has trained us to set high standards for our pleasures, as though God had better come up with a million dollar budget for props or the scene won't be worth watching.

"Exciting" and "captivating" have come to mean "true," like those flashy commercials designed to convince us that Coca Cola is "The Real Thing." (For a beverage that full of artificial, non-nutritive chemicals and artificial bubbles, it's hardly what I would call even "a" real thing.) Ordinary life pales by comparison with the media hype we take for granted. So I'll warn you now: according to that standard, subtle perception may at first seem pale.

When was the last time you took a walk outside on a clear night to go stargazing? It can be such a contrast to go from your living room, with its bright electricity, to the natural lighting under the sky. The deeper into the country you go, the longer it takes to accustom yourself to the darkness. And the more you eventually see.

Once your eyes adjust to the subtle frequencies, there's a beauty to those pinpoints of ethereal silver. Sure they don't beat upon your senses like Technicolor on a high-tech screen. But the sight of the stars feels realer. It stirs the soul.

This is the kind of flash that comes when you connect with auras, a kind of inner Aha! It may come through vision or another sense. After all, the loveliest moonlight walk is more than a pretty picture.

Which is the best part for you? Could it be the hush over a stilled landscape, the texture of moon-dusted air against your cheeks, the fragrance of sleeping earth and starlight?

Even if you're sure that the sight of the stars alone is what makes you go "Ahh," what aspect of vision does it? Do you thrill to the mere light itself or is it a feeling that the sight of the stars could springboard you into other worlds, if the rest of you only knew how to follow?

Whichever way you connect with the magic of a starry night, that is your inner truth, the truth your perception is set up to find. Others may have a truth that sounds more intriguing. Need that make it better than yours?

No one human being can lay claim to the definitive inner truth. That fact applies to aura reading as well as to any other subjective knowledge.

The Element of Trust

By now you appreciate that auras are perceived outwardly but experienced inwardly. Also, inward experience is, by definition, *subtle*. If you don't pay close, caring attention, you'll miss it.

Add to this one other fact and you, the aspiring aura reader, come up against a gigantic challenge. And that other fact is that **aura reading is a spiritual experience**. It is not physical, literal, outwardly obvious.

Meaning? Nobody else can convey to you what it is like to have direct experience of the subtle. Therefore, your willingness to explore auras requires an openmindedness so great, you could call it a leap of spiritual trust.

Those who already read auras do what they can to awaken this trust. Clairvoyants commission paintings. Scientists display Kirlian photographs. Dowsers use rods. Sometimes aura readers impress skeptics through use of a pendulum.

I can get into the act too. Occasionally I've dangled a pendulum in front of a skeptic's aura. Tea bags work well. (You use the kind that hangs by a string from a little paper tag. And, yes, that's a fresh, dry tea bag.) Position the bag a few inches from the aura's main centers (you'll read about them later). Allow the pendulum to hang without interference from you. Voila! The energy field will cause the pendulum to move in ways that show patterns of auric energy.

Sometimes I give demonstrations in other ways, too. For instance, I'll use my hands to point out the size of the aura over different parts of the body. I can go on to describe what the aura communicates—plenty of detail about the individual's emotional life, ability to communicate, sense of personal power. Teenage girls squeal when I read this.

"My God, it's so true!" "This is really incredible."

"Not so incredible really," I'll answer.

It's an established scientific fact that we have electromagnetic fields all around our physical forms. In metaphysical terms, these are auras.

Each person has several subtle bodies that overlap like the layers of an onion... but sweeter. And each of these subtle bodies, or layers, can be read.

Given how packed auras are with layer upon layer of information, the incredible thing would be if auras told us nothing.

For extra impact, when clients are game, I will use subtle hearing to sing out auric patterns—sounds like chuckling, carbonation, mutters, grumbles, and tones that ascend up, up, up.

Admittedly these efforts to communicate have some flash. They grab attention. Moderate skeptics turn into moderate believers. Believers say, "Tell me what to do. I want to start NOW."

But even at their best, demonstrations are merely signs and symbols. Only *you* can give yourself the genuine article. That's the purpose of this book's aforementioned hundred tips and techniques. Only you can supply the trust to give them a chance.

Underlying Beliefs—
Yours and Mine

What must you believe in order to be able to read auras? Aura reading is not, in itself, the exclusive property of any religion. Nor should aura reading conflict with your religion. Pictures of Jesus, Buddha, Krishna, and other spiritual luminaries often include a glowing aura around the head. Why not learn to read it?

Regardless of whether or not you practice a formal religion, you must be willing to approach auras as something spiritual to feel comfortable with the approach to aura reading in this particular book. Not all aura reading is presented this way. I couldn't help it. I'm a mystic, a long-time spiritual explorer. Disguising my approach is out of the question. To me, auras are spiritual.

Must that leave science out? Not necessarily. To the extent that you believe in science as a touchstone for truth, you can consider aura reading as a kind of research into consciousness.

Note this, however: Some important pioneers in making aura reading acceptable to a skeptical public, such as Barbara Brennan, author of *Hands of Light*, and Rosalyn Bruyere, author of *Wheels of Light*, have labored hard to standardize subtle perception for scientific research. Consequently, for them, the measure of a student's success is the extent to which that student develops perceptions that match the teacher's.

But this teacher's approach couldn't be more different. My intent is to help you develop your own celestial perception, not copy mine. Therefore, I measure any student's success—that means yours!—by these three things:

1. Naturalness

It's natural to read auras. Do your perceptions come easily, without inner struggle?

2. Recognition

Do your aura readings resonate for you as truth?

To be aware of this sort of resonance, you must learn to trust and listen deeply to your own experience—something you may have learned long before you picked up this book. With practice at inner listening, you come to recognize that your truth has a familiar quality. You could call it *feeling true, golden wisdom, the still small voice within, Aha!, resonance.* Call it whatever you like and know that aura readings can bring it to you every time.

3. Helpfulness

Successful aura readings prove helpful to others as well as yourself. The proof of the pudding is in the eating. When the pudding is subtle, expect results to be subtle, subtle but noticeable.

In short, the approach to aura reading you'll find here is spiritual and subjective. One-size-fits all evidence is not the goal. The goal is for you to discover, trust, and live from a deeper level of truth. It's a higher state of consciousness you'll read more about later, celestial consciousness.

Spiritual seekers yearn for this kind of experience. Why should it stay a dream? Claim it for your everyday reality.

Chapter 2

Discover the Truth about Auras

ura *Reading Through All Your Senses* presents a unique approach to developing subtle perception. Mostly this book consists of experiments. You explore what interests you and draw conclusions accordingly.

This chapter is different though. It consists of ideas, pure and simple and sometimes mind boggling. The new experience of aura reading demands a new framework of understanding.

For example, how can you use your sensing gifts to the fullest until you know what these gifts are? Probably you have more talents for perception than you think you do. Let's find out.

The Myth about Auras

If you put a paper bag over your head, how well do you think you'd see auras?

Not very well, you say? The funny thing is, most of us have worn that paper bag for years. This limitation has been brought to you courtesy of humanity's collective fantasies, fears, power struggles, and downright ignorance.

Like other prejudices passed from one generation to another, false ideas have blinded us to the true nature of subtle perception. Sure we've learned about gross physical reality, the one-size-fits-all perception that comes in so handy for communicating with each other. We've learned to look at a face, identify the eyes, nose, and mouth. But how about the energy pulsating around that face?

Here's where you need to use subtle perception. Turning it on is like allowing yourself to fall in love. It makes you vulnerable. It helps you grow. It takes trust.

Unfortunately, most of us "know" too much. We label and move on, which means we lose out. That's why the first step in aura reading is to un-learn the myth about auras. How many of the following statements can you vaguely recognize from some deep corner of your subconscious mind? How many do you consciously believe?

1. Auras are colors around people that gifted ones SEE—seeing is the only way to read an aura.

2. Someone who claims to read auras without seeing them does not get the whole truth, compared with someone who *can* see them.

3. Seeing auras means that, wherever you look, you see colors around people.

4. Each of these colors means something specific and...

5. A good teacher of aura reading tells you what each color means.

6. People who see auras are spiritually gifted;

7. Being better at aura reading than the rest of us, they should be looked up to as authorities, the ones who decide if other people's readings are valid.

8. Talent for aura reading always makes itself known during childhood.

9. When (and if) I ever become spiritually enlightened, auras will be switched on for me, too.

10. Aura readers all see the same thing and understand it the same way.

11. Thus, aura readers are like members of a club who all know a secret password. They observe a hidden reality unavailable to the rest of us.

The Truth about Auras

1. Let's start with a definition of auras. They are far more than "colors," just as people are far more than what they physically look like. Auras are energy fields, subtle bodies that wrap around the physical body. Accordingly, auras are packed with layer upon layer of information: what is going on with a person's emotions, health, and spiritual development.

Auras show influences from the past, a complete array of information about the present, even tendencies that can be projected into the future.

> **Unlike body language, expression, and other aspects**
> **of a person that can be manipulated**
> **to give a desired appearance, auras can't be faked—**
> **one more reason why they are useful to read.**

As for auras being something whose truth only shows in what is seen, that's ridiculous! Have you ever had somebody judge your worth based entirely on your physical looks? It doesn't seem fair because it isn't. Even Miss America Contests aren't run that way any more. As for auras, like people, they are far more complex than they look.

2. When it comes to "the" whole truth about an aura, no one human being can claim to know it. That's because perception of auras is spiritual, not literal. In spiritual matters, the best a human being can do is to know his or her whole truth: the most complete and honest set of information, recognized in the ways that are personally most meaningful.

By analogy, if you were praying, would it be your business to compose "the" perfect prayer for everyone? Your job, my job, is to pray our own prayers. Let other people pray theirs. Well, the same goes for subtle perception.

To find your whole truth of perception, it helps to know that there are at least 11 ways to "see" auras. All these forms of subtle perception are connected, at their core, through the principle of *synesthesia* (pronounced sin-ess-THEE-zha).

A dictionary definition of synesthesia is that "one type of stimulation evokes the sensation of another, as the hearing of a sound resulting in the sensation of the visualization of a color."

A practical definition of synesthesia is, simply, the senses working together.

Just because your senses work together doesn't mean that everyone has the same order of preference among the senses. Not at all! Research into learning styles has documented a variety of forms of intelligence. For instance, according to the authors of *How Your Child Is Smart*, Dawna Markova, Ph.D., and Anne R. Powell, the primary sense for knowing your whole truth could be hearing, touch, or sight. All senses are equally valid.

> **As an aura reader, it's best to emphasize the sense**
> **that comes to you most easily. This sense will help you**
> **find your way in to a deeper level**
> **for perceiving through all your senses.**
> **Use of your other subtle senses will follow automatically.**

3. Even when perception of auras is visual, colors may not be involved. Your subtle sight can appear in different forms, such as light (colored or not), patterns of energy, even knowledge that comes as a result of looking but involves no visual flash at all.

4. To teach that an auric color like yellow—or any subtle perception—must mean one thing for everyone is worse than wrong. Set meanings tempt people to strain or pretend, then interpret their perceptions according to someone else's pattern; thus they miss *their* unique ability to know truth.

5. Many teachers do push their personal *aura reading dictionary* as though it were gospel. That's how they develop a following. But is that what *you* need in a teacher?

   Instead you can choose to accept a teacher as guide but consider yourself to be the ultimate authority on your celestial perception. More power to you for having such spiritual spunk! You will discover that you have a unique *inner dictionary*. It flows out of your built-in strengths of subtle perception and connects to the spiritual work that only you can do.

6. Everyone is spiritually gifted. So everyone can perceive and interpret auras. Nevertheless, we don't all have one identical gift. As you become an aura reader, a big part of the fun will be discovering and developing your own gifts.

7. Are people who can read auras better than people who can't (yet)? No. Do they have access to more information? Yes. But how they use it is up to them. Beware anyone who uses aura reading as a means to claim superiority.

8. The timing for unfoldment of your celestial perception is part of the perfect story of your personal evolution. No one timing is superior. If you're interested enough in auras to read this book, you're ready now, whether you're eight or eighty.

9. Most people must actively switch on their subtle perception and interpretation. No matter how high a level of consciousness you may attain, it will remain true that you must make a choice to pay attention to auras. But the choice to switch-on is easy. Your personal gates of perception are set up to open without struggle or strain. Just ask.

10. The funniest way to prove that aura readers perceive differently is to compare the color pictures in books by clairvoyants. Their "definitive" versions contradict each other like crazy. Nevertheless, each system works—for the clairvoyant who developed it.

You, too, can develop a system of aura reading that works perfectly. Just don't make the mistake of calling it "The One True System for Everyone."

11. Some clairvoyants give the impression that aura readers form a club of interchangeable psychics. Authentic spirituality is different; don't worry about joining a club.

**External validation is the wrong direction
to look for spiritual truth.**

Hidden realities are available to you, to seek and to share. What you experience privately, the way God made you, is the contribution you alone can make to spiritual wisdom.

Five Subtle Senses

The human senses are physical. Yet artists, lovers, and mystics throughout the ages have learned a deeper truth about the senses: they are also spiritual. **Your senses can lead you to bliss, if only your perception goes deep enough.**

Here are the relevant spiritual facts of life.

1. Your perception through any sense contains levels of increasing subtlety, nested like Russian dolls.

2. Synesthesia means that all your senses are interconnected at the subtlest of these levels, the celestial level.

3. To experience at a level so close to the Creator is to connect with *bliss*, a concentrated form of spiritual joy.

4. The more you develop your subtle perception through any one sense, the more easily synesthesia will enliven your perception through other subtle senses.

What makes the concept of subtle senses vitally important is that you have at least one of them available to you right now. It is a gift, a spiritual pathway open to you for experiencing at the subtlest level of all your senses. So far you may not have recognized that you have any perceptual gifts at all. So the first step is to understand what they are.

The following descriptions will give you a working definition of the most common subtle senses. Some of the descriptions will jump out at you. Pay attention! Later chapters of this book will give you opportunities to explore the gifts that are already lively for you and help you develop the others. Check the Glossary for definitions along the way.

1. Clairvoyance

To Joyce, imagination means visualization, making pictures. Visions are so commonplace, they're no big deal to her. In fact, the only thing Joyce would have real trouble picturing is how life would be if she were blind.

Not all natural clairvoyants share Joyce's gift for visions. Others find they can effortlessly remember faces and visual details. (Sure, nonclairvoyants can train themselves to do this too, but why bother? It's easier for them to remember people through other subtle senses instead.)

Color is tremendously important to people with subtle sight; the stronger your clairvoyance, the deeper the impact of every hue. To non-clairvoyants, color is incidental or maybe not noticed at all. But if you have been put together as strongly visual, color strikes you constantly. It's a major aspect of clothing and home furnishings. It's everywhere. Color has meaning for you, reaching right to your core.

Do you catch yourself throughout the day doing makeovers on people? Or rooms? Maybe you wonder why most folks don't do a better job of presenting themselves. Answer: They're not strong on subtle sight.

But here's consolation if you find visual tackiness seriously annoying. Your irritation proves that you care passionately, which shows you should explore clairvoyance. And by using this to create beauty you can trigger your sense of rightness in the world.

Of all people, clairvoyants are most likely to see auras in color. Sometimes colors come spontaneously, unsought. Such perceptions seem to raise more questions than they answer. If this has been your experience, relax. Techniques in this book will help you expand your gift for subtle sight, along with skill at consulting your inner dictionary. This combination will empower you to master the art of aura reading.

2. Clairsentience

With clairsentience, information comes along with touch. Rosa, for instance, is a massage therapist. When starting a session, Rosa holds her client by the ankles. Information comes to her about what needs work. It's as though the body reveals its secrets to her hands.

Some people with this gift come across as very physical and sexy. They may not realize the extent to which *physical* touching brings information that is *subtle.* On the other hand, as it were, some subtle touchers can seem unconcerned with their own physicality. Subtle perception is so much more interesting than staying in touch with "reality."

Here's another paradox. Clairsentient people work especially well with their hands, for example, in writing, cooking, or gardening. But ask them if they like to work with their hands and they may well say "No." How come?

It's one of those mind-stopping Zen trains of thought, like explaining the sound of one hand clapping. Why don't some clairsentients notice their hands? The process of creating through the hands is so charming it totally absorbs their attention. Therefore, what part of the mind is left to notice the hands?

As a clairsentient, whether you come across as grounded or more of an absent-minded professor, you know the value of hugging and touching. That's how you feel you have made genuine contact with people. And if your clairsentience goes along with a gift for physical healing, your hands may radiate a special spiritual beauty.

3. Clairaudience

Milton says he can't carry a tune. But if you play any note on the piano he can tell you what it is. Perfect pitch helps him play the double bass. In fact, Milton has been a famous jazz musician for years.

Clairaudients notice nuances of hearing, though perfect pitch is rare, even among them. If you're strong in subtle hearing, the right music can soothe you, even transport you. Whether or not you make the music yourself doesn't figure into this, incidentally. Mastering an instrument takes coordination, physical and psychological endowments, plus a good teacher. Clairaudients need not be performers in the outer world for their perception to be subtle.

As part of subtle hearing, clairaudients appreciate nuances of silence. (The flip side is that unpleasant noises will get to you too.) Think about your ideal work environment. Does it come complete with very specific requirements for the sound in the background? Then count natural clairaudience as one of your gifts.

As a *trained* clairaudient, you will pick up information through inner hearing of words; maybe you will inwardly listen to music from planes beyond the physical, detecting tones that emanate from people and places. Clairaudients can be sensitive to resonance, too. For example, Eric is a successful professional speaker and trainer. He changed my life when he gave me this tip:

"The most important thing when you speak to an audience," he said, "is to listen for the hollow echo."

"What's that?" I asked.

"When your audience stops listening to you, your voice begins to carry a different sound. There's a deadness, as though the sound waves bounce right back to you instead of going out to the people. When you hear that hollow echo, stop. Shake up the people or you've lost them."

Still wondering whether or not you're clairaudient? The bottom line may be that you recognize people by their voices, their accents, or their speech patterns. (Sorry, that doesn't mean you're necessarily better than non-clairaudients at remembering strangers by name.)

4. Emotional Touch

Bruce's friends joke that he's scary. You can't get away with a thing. Silent anger, holding a grudge—forget it. Bruce always knows what you're feeling.

For those who share his gift, emotional touch comes as naturally as breathing. In fact, even a routine activity like hearing somebody breathe can tell you emotional secrets. Whatever the means of your probing, you pick up the person's underlying feeling state just about anywhere. Sounds of breathing, expressions on a face, the smell of a meal, any one of these turns you into an emotional Sherlock Holmes.

People who live more in their heads may criticize you for responding emotionally to most situations. So what? What does a little social embarrassment matter compared to the added juice in all your relationships? Wherever you put your attention—on others' actions or your own—you can find an emotion and learn from it.

Those gifted in this way are often emotional risk takers. How far do you extend yourself to others? Do you ask questions that others wouldn't dare ask? When in the company of people who are plodding along, emotionally stuck, do you find yourself compelled to stir things up?

Count it as subtle perception. You recognize at a deep level when a person is emotionally stuck. Someone without your gift might overlook the dead space. Thanks to your gift, you can tell the emotionally quick from the dead—also from the peaceful, the inward, the resisting, and the half-asleep.

And on the subject of emotional variety, do those with emotional touch thrill to soap operas, the more dramatically lurid the better? Highly unlikely. Life, in living emotional color, is sensational enough.

5. Gustatory Giftedness

Audrey has an unusual problem. When crowded together with many people on a bus or at the movies, the smells drive her crazy. To her it's a nightmare of clashing odors: perfumes, aftershaves, hair products, and sweat.

Audrey is so gifted, she could be a professional nose for the fragrance industry. But many equally talented sniffers do not suffer at all. Their blessing comes unmixed as smell and taste trigger layer upon layer of information.

Do you love to read about food? Can you mentally taste a dish just by thinking about it? Then you've passed one test for being gustatorily (goose-ta-TOR-uh-lee) gifted.

Here's another possibility. Do you pick up on the vibes of the cook? Makes the dining experience a bit more intense, doesn't it? Recommended reading is Laura Esquivel's *Like Water For Chocolate*, a novel that mingles emotions and taste. This fiction confirms by exaggeration how food picks up subtle flavors corresponding to a cook's happiness, seductiveness, bragging, boredom, and so forth.

Fast food Happy Meals may not taste tremendously happy to you, when you consciously chomp on the vibes of the food handlers. An interesting exercise for you with *trained* gustatory gifts plus subtle sight will be to taste the energy of your food, then look around the restaurant to observe energy changes in the auras of other diners.

Another way where your nose for subtle news can come into play is healing. During sessions of healing or meditation, you may notice a fragrance that isn't necessarily physically present. Should gardenias fill the room, don't feel you must either track down the incense or doubt your sanity. Instead congratulate yourself on gustatory giftedness.

In essence, this gift means that smell and taste trigger your awareness of spiritual flavors. These flavors don't have to be physical. Every experience or idea can match up with a quality or flavor. When Newton was hit on the head with an apple, his Aha! had a flavor. And probably it expressed a different quality than ordinary applesauce.

Sixth Sense (s)

Here are more subtle faculties of knowing. Each could be called a sixth sense. They don't relate directly to one of the physical senses; instead they result from the soul's connectedness to planes beyond earth. Unless you're metaphysically minded, this idea could strike you as hopelessly abstract or even outrageous. Keep an open mind, though. What matters is what your own sixth sense (or senses) can tell you?

> **Undoubtedly you have had past experience of these mysterious forms of perception. As you read through the following descriptions, think about how they may apply to yourself and to other people you know.**

1. Emotional Empathy

Sally can't stop crying. She's been crying all morning because her mother feels sad but can't express it. Neither woman knows the reason for what is happening with Sally.

It's not unusual. Most natural empaths do not know they are empaths. This gift goes far beyond the perceptiveness described earlier as emotional touch. With empathy, someone else's emotional data becomes your personal experience. You slip into it so effortlessly, you don't even know you're doing it—at least not until you become a skilled empath rather than, simply, a natural empath.

Natural, unskilled emotional empathy is, frankly, a mixed blessing. Sure, you have a priceless gift for service to others. Unfortunately, your inner life is probably tempestuous, due to constantly taking on other people's emotional stuff. The trick to becoming a skilled empath is to notice how your gift works, including how to switch the empathy button off or on at will. Instructions for turning off *unwelcome perception* will be discussed in a later chapter.

Also helpful will be this book's explanations about how to interpret your subtle perception. Finally, aura reading with senses other than emotional empathy will help you to become most balanced and productive as an empath.

2. Physical Empathy

Zap! With physical empathy, another person's physical sensations become your own. For example, imagine feeling Jeff's headache inside your own skull. All it takes to trigger this, if you are an unskilled physical empath, is being in the same room with Jeff, a person whose body needs healing. Much as some people can catch a yawn from each other, a physical empath can temporarily catch another person's aches and pains.

Another version of physical empathy is, literally, "I know how you feel." The empath's consciousness slides right into Jeff's body, feeling the headache as though inside Jeff's head. This experience can be triggered by any one of the five subtle senses described in the previous section: watching Jeff, hearing the sound of his voice, shaking his hand, noticing the odor of his body, imagining how food tastes to him.

Physical empathy from "I know how you feel" could even be a springboard to soul travel. (For more thorough exploration of subtle senses as a means to *soul travel*, see the book about Eckankar in the Bibliography.)

But the trouble with any kind of physical empathy, when natural rather than skilled, is that the empath doesn't consciously know what he's doing. Instead he carries a lot of physical sensations, many of them disturbing. I remember asking one natural empath, "Are you sick all the time or do you just think you're a hypochondriac?"

"Just a hypochondriac," she laughed. Emily was in her fifties, well educated and psychologically astute. A lavish upper class lifestyle had given her many advantages in life, but until our conversation she didn't have a clue about what empathy was or that she had it.

> **Auras of empaths move in a distinctive, recognizable way—recognizable, at least, if noticing empathy in others is part of *your* spiritual gift as an aura reader. When you spot empaths, you can do them a big favor by educating them about their gift.**

Should you be the one who is a physical empath, it's going to give you a big advantage in life to learn to handle it. For instance, here's how Mark used to "cheat" in gymnastics class as a kid. The teacher would describe how to do a particular stunt, then demonstrate. Instead of following the teacher's instructions, Mark would mentally put himself inside the teacher's body during the demonstration. Knowing how the teacher felt, Mark would duplicate the feeling. His body would follow through by doing the new stunt perfectly. Some short cut that would be for most of us!

3. Analytical Awareness

For John Paul's entire adult life, friends have urged him to move out of his head and into his feelings. But why? Because that's how *they* function best?

If you're like John Paul, analytical awareness is the key to your most subtle and powerful perceptions. God forbid you should move away! Analyzing shows you a deeper truth, and that's what you live for. What lies beneath the surface? What's underneath that?

Analytical awareness is the subtle sense of mental agility. To a far greater extent than for people lacking this gift, perception comes through the mind. Therefore, this sense exposes levels of understanding so fine that most people could not hold onto them consciously.

Here's where recognizing the gift of analytical awareness becomes tricky. Most people believe that they intellectually travel from layer to layer, but really they stay stuck on one layer of truth, from there entertaining *ideas* about other layers. Only those with analytical awareness really do the genuine mental hopscotch, deftly leaping from layer to layer.

The best example may come from music. Baroque music buffs, did you ever wonder what goes on in the minds of musicians who play Bach organ works? Two or three or more musical lines interweave at the same time, each line being a complete and highly complex world of musical expression. Could anyone who plays music like that *not* have analytical awareness? Unlikely.

With a gift like this, you thrive on complexity. Nobody sees more layers to life than you. It's a priceless intellectual treasure.

For aura reading purposes, though, analytical awareness is the trickiest gift to handle. Used correctly, analytical awareness can position your mind precisely in the direction for going after a certain kind of auric information. But you still have to let go of all meaning and plunge into the subtle experience, vague and unformulated though it appears.

So keep this in mind if you are analytically aware: When you do techniques for aura reading, subtle perception is not simply one more concept to play with. Auras are an experience, to which you can later supply appropriate understanding, so long as you save that mental analysis for *after* you do your readings. Ideas are no substitute for direct experience.

4. Holistic Knowing

Mary is such a connector—of people, of skills, of ideas. Some acquaintances see her as a social butterfly, even a dilettante. Do they ever miss the point! Mary appreciates things from a very deep level. Do you share her gift for holistic knowing? Then you, too, feel an incomparable thrill from making a creative connection within yourself or facilitating that connection for others.

Holistic knowing can involve *holding a space* (in consciousness) (see Glossary) big enough for a variety of people or ideas to harmonize, however briefly.

For instance, Mary's favorite aspect of teaching elementary school is balancing the strengths and weaknesses of her students, finding elegant use for every possible human resource. To do this, she holds a space for each of the students.

"Why don't my kids' teachers figure out how to use everyone together? It's the best part of the job." she complained to me once. How could I convince Mary how unusual it is for a teacher—or anyone—to have the high degree of holistic awareness that Mary takes for granted?

Making holistic connections is a kind of spiritual recycling. Every linkage brings joy, and joy brings new common denominators that have nothing to do with logic. Still, in holistic terms, they work.

In everyday life, holistic knowing is often the basis for *telepathy*, the spiritual ability to merge consciousness with another intelligence. Telepathy brings knowledge that can be used in practical ways. (However, as is true for any spiritual experience, the degree of clarity for the perceiver is inversely proportional to the amount of ego involvement. Use the gift for selfish ends and it will fade away.)

One benefit of holistic knowing for aura reading is that it includes a strong intuitive understanding of synesthesia. Why shouldn't you appreciate that senses are connected at their deepest level when, on a daily basis, you turn up one interrelationship after another? By welcoming synesthesia, you smooth the way for rapid development of one subtle sense after another.

Another benefit of holistic knowing for aura reading is that you're a natural for appreciating how people affect each other energetically. (Be sure to read about *group body* in Chapter Four.)

5. Truth Knowledge

When Wyatt did the exercise on seeing people's auras (coming up for you in a later chapter), he wasn't aware of seeing a thing but empty space. Yet very specific thoughts came to him, like: "Joe's favorite color is blue," and "Lately he has been eating too many hamburgers for his own good, which he is aware of but prefers to ignore."

What a perfect demonstration of truth knowledge. This intuitive gift takes you directly to your destination, like a no-frills airline. You just know. That doesn't mean you know how you know; you simply *know*. Frustration arises when you demand a flashy experience to justify your knowledge.

Back at the example of Wyatt's aura reading, his perception bypassed sensory symbols, going directly to truth at the subtlest level of senses, the *seed form* (see Glossary).

Truth knowledge means you know how to *read the seed*. This may seem "weird" to people whose trust of information rises in direct proportion to how literal it appears to be. They would prefer Wyatt's reading to sound more like this:

"Joe's aura displays a swirl of turquoise over his left shoulder, which means that his favorite color is blue. His aura also pictures a half-eaten Big Mac floating in a grey cloud over the solar plexus, signifying overindulgence in animal products."

A reading like this could be fine, but so is Wyatt's. Truth knowledge, short and sweet, is a perfectly valid form of subtle perception.

6. Psychic Knowing

Joanna was awakened in the middle of the night by an earthquake, long distance. For several hours she shared the physical and emotional experiences of hundreds of people involved in the quake. Next morning Joanna heard a news report of the disaster, which had occurred in California. Meanwhile Joanna's physical body had been sleeping in Maryland.

That's trained psychic knowing for you. The gift works like truth knowledge, physical empathy, and emotional empathy all rolled into one—and definitely available long distance. When knowledge comes, you experience the auras of people far away in time and space. Not only that—the information may feel up close and personal.

As a teacher, I have found two different situations where people have dramatic experiences of psychic knowing. Sometimes the knower is like Joanna. Vivid though her experiences may be, they don't overwhelm her because:

- She has worked for years to develop her subtle perception through regular practice.
- Lifestyle choices keep her in excellent physical and emotional health.
- Her personal life is in balance. Spiritual service represents only one part of a balanced life.
- She has consciously chosen to use her spiritual gifts for service.

The second situation seems more like a spiritual wakeup call and sometimes it can be downright scary. Psychic knowing drops like a bombshell into the home of someone who has ignored less dramatic invitations to become aware of spiritual life.

For instance, Frank is a yuppie who works in advertising. His life abounds with pleasures and pressures. So it took an intense experience of psychic knowing to grab his attention.

Soul to Frank: *Would you please make some time in your busy life for me? For God?*

Aura reading does not necessarily involve psychic knowing. Nor do all aura readers wish to get involved with it. However, if you would like to develop this form of sensing, use a variation of the inner dictionary technique, as described in Chapter Three.

Altogether you have now had a chance to identify eleven different abilities for subtle perception. What jumped out at you? Did you recognize some of your major gifts? Remember, *one* subtle sense is all you need to open the doors to perception.

Affirm Your Right to Know the Truth about Auras

Your preparation to start reading auras is nearly complete. Now it's time for one last step.

As a result of my teaching aura reading and related abilities to thousands of students over the past 25 years, I've found that most people, consciously or unconsciously, carry inner resistance to using intuition fully. Affirmation, the verbal declaration of spiritual truth, can go a long way toward removing this resistance. The following affirmation was developed to clear your path.

To benefit most, begin by reading through the words silently. Alter the language until it fits you like a glove. Then speak the affirmation out loud.

You may wish to copy your affirmation onto an index card and carry it with you for a while, repeating it many times a day to saturate your subconscious mind:

I am a spiritual being, made in the image of God and

filled with the presence of God.

I have the right to use every one of my God-given gifts. No

other person, or group of people, has the right to limit

me spiritually. I am the authority in my life.

I release all fear of knowing a deeper truth. My desire to

know is stronger than any old patterns of fear. I am

worthy to receive my full celestial perception.

I will use it only for good. At every step of my spiritual

path, God protects me.

Therefore I am ready to receive the deepest knowledge

appropriate to me at this time.

Chapter 3

Engage the Energy

As my friends at the gym might say: "Okay, gang. Let's lift some vibes!" Every time you read an aura, you engage the energy of spiritual life. Vibrationally you are lifted. By virtue of a sincere desire to know truth, you can open your senses, heart, and mind to a magical beauty deep within life.

Regardless of how seriously you take the prospect of reading auras, this chapter can help you move forward. I've packed this chapter with exercises to develop your celestial perception. For best results with each of these experiments, please read through all the steps first. Afterwards turn to the Question and Answer (Q&A) section.

This special Q&A format is my way of bringing you into a workshop where you can join in spirit with other new aura readers, sharing the struggles and joys of opening up new subtle sense abilities. **Please remember to be kind to yourself as you do the exercises. After all, you are doing the spiritual equivalent of learning to walk.** It brings a deep down thrill, as though Independence Day fireworks are just starting; unexpected light is exploding over a deep indigo sky. Only this time, the colors that burst into shimmering form will be happening within you. Like the most beautiful fireworks display, however, this show starts small before it bursts into light. So be patient. Your inner light show may not be as flashy as the outer kind requiring gunpowder. Still, there's this advantage: once switched on, your aura reading won't be over in half an hour, either. It can last a lifetime.

Aura Bounce

Meet and greet the auric energy coming out of your hands. Remember to start by reading through the steps that follow. Do them one by one. Only then turn to the Q&A.

1. Sit comfortably in a chair, nothing in your lap or hands.

2. Turn your hands into a tool for subtle perception. Cup your hands, as if you were about to hold water in them. Separate them, still keeping fingers and thumbs drawn close to the palm. Voila! You have created two compact energy-catching mitts. From now on, they will be referred to as *hands in sensor position*. Use this position throughout the aura bounce.

3. Hold your hands apart, shoulder width. Clap them together. Separate them. Clap twice more, each time more slowly.

4. Now comes the interesting part: Continue clapping in slow motion but be aware that, located somewhere between your hands (before they physically touch), you can feel a blob of energy.

5. Soon as you feel it, stop. Then draw back a few inches and approach the energy with smaller motions. This enables you to pat the edges as you would firm up a snowball.

6. The energy you're feeling comes from your own aura as it radiates outward from each hand. Notice how much energy there is. Experiment by bouncing in various ways:

   - Bring hands together faster.

- Bring hands together super slowly. (Remember to keep hands in sensor position; it will weaken your experience if energy "leaks" out through your fingers.)

- Bounce with your eyes closed.

- Do an occasional goofy bounce, where your hands miss each other entirely and whack the air instead. Does it feel different, empty?

7. Doubts and questions may come up. Lay them aside to deal with later. For now, play in the energy. If you must give your mind something to ponder, ask it this:

How far out do I feel this aura go?

Aura Bounce

Q. **What was that stuff?**

A. That was your aura.

Q. **How do you know it wasn't heat or sweat or radiation or something else?**

A. You don't. There are many levels to explain most things in life, but what we're paying attention to now is the level of aura.

Q. **Was it okay that my energy felt prickly? I did the aura bounce with some friends, and they used words like "hot" and "soft." Could my aura be strange, or did I just describe it wrong?**

A. Everything you did was right except comparing yourself to other people. Think back to what you have read about how "Each person has a unique dictionary." How you perceive, the words you use, it's all very personal.

Sex is my favorite analogy for the experience of subtle perception. When your partner embraces you passionately, do you say this?

"Stop everything. Before we kiss any more we must make sure that both of us feel exactly the same thing. Unless we use identical words to describe it, I can't be sure that this is really sex."

Maybe the kiss seems "urgently hot" to him while it strikes you as "meltingly, irresistibly tingly." Problem? To have the deepest experience of sex, let yourself go with whatever turns you on. In the same way, for the deepest experience of subtle perception, go with what turns you on.

Q. **Nice analogy but doesn't it break down regarding words? Words may not be necessary for sex but aura readers must need to develop language for that inner dictionary you talk about.**

A. True. Giving an aura reading means that you have a subtle perception, then interpret it through the aid of your inner dictionary. "Prickly" is the word for you to remember because you'll be looking it up later. Your inner dictionary will have a listing for the words that occur to you spontaneously, not necessarily for the words that others use.

Q. **I didn't feel anything. What did I do wrong?**

A. Expecting, probably. Please set expectations aside. Especially don't expect a sensation so gross that it hits you over the head. We're talking about subtle perception, right?

If you're stuck, here's your prescription: Do more bounces today, in different moods and settings. By the end of the day you'll probably sneak past your resistance. If not, skip ahead to the exercise called "Mirror Technique." Finish the rest of this chapter, then loop back to here.

Q. **I just tried again. I think maybe I felt something with my hands about two inches apart. Was that the right distance?**

A. Sure, that was right for this time. No one right distance applies to everyone or even to the same person every time.

Q. **Could you give me a range?**

A. My goodness, you must be an engineer! All right, anywhere from half an inch apart to four feet ... usually. But please don't measure. Just go for where the energy feels strongest. Analytical awareness can be a subtle sense but right now you're using it to stay on the surface level.

You're better off closing your eyes and turning off your mind. Bounce your hands at different rates of speed. Experiment. Don't worry. Your mind will be there when you need it. Later.

Q. **But thinking about things always helps me do better. Look, I went to college. I'm a professional. I am an engineer! Why are you telling me not to think?**

A. Auras aren't about thinking. They are about direct perception. Suspend your disbelief. Switch on your subtle senses.

Later you'll be able to put your experiences into an elegant system. But you must let yourself have them first.

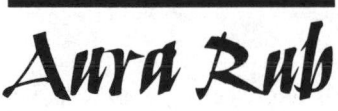

Now that you've met your aura, how about making deeper contact? As always, start by reading all the way through the steps of an exercise. Do them one by one. Only then turn to the Q&A.

1. Cup your hands in sensor position, palms facing and shoulder width apart. Bounce your hands back and forth until you get to the point where you feel energy.

2. Move your hands a bit closer together (though still not physically touching). This means reaching inside your aura. Now rub your hands back and forth, gently, to feel the energy.

Why rub? It's as though you were sitting in a comfortable bath. Once adjusted to the temperature, you wouldn't notice it unless you swished the water around a bit. Similarly, your aura is so familiar you need to stir it up to notice it. How does the energy feel?

3. Explore with eyes closed, then again with eyes open.

4. Describe this blob of energy in words. Is it hard? Soft? Springy? Spongy? Does it have temperature, texture?

Aura Rub

Q. **My aura felt hot, amazingly hot. How do I know if what I felt was genuine?**

A. Were you expecting it to be hot?

Q. **No ....**

A. Why else would you have had the perception, unless it were genuine?

Q. **I wish my energy could be described by something simple, the way hers was hot—**

A. Oops, no comparing yourself to others allowed! Start again, please.

Q. **My energy did feel different this time, compared to the aura bounce. But I don't have the words to describe it. Does something that sloppy count?**

A. Sure. Here's how to refine it: the next few times you do the aura rub, put your hands into the energy and *playfully* try out words to describe what you feel. To loosen up your awareness, purposely include words that seem totally ridiculous.

Q. **Like shivery, lumpy, purple—**
Hey, it did feel kind of purple. How can a touch feel like a color?

A. That's synesthesia. Remember, perception through any one sense links up at the deepest level to all the other senses. Usually adults are "educated" to sort the senses into strict categories, but you'll hear kids say things like "My jacket is too yellow. The color tickles my eyes," or "That cookie tastes really loud."

Some grownups have managed to retain their ability to experience the senses in terms of each other. For example, I've heard that Tchaikovsky used synesthesia when he wrote The Nutcracker. Everyone can rediscover synesthesia; aura reading can help.

Q. **Perception-wise I'm definitely in the clairsentient category. If I develop my synesthesia, will I eventually *see* auras by touching them?**

A. Yes. And that's one reason why it's silly to value seeing over the other senses. Start out using your strongest modality of perception. This will bring you to deep levels of subtle sensing, where you have synesthesia. From there, you can branch out to all the other senses.

Aura Handshake

Here's your first interpersonal technique to develop subtle touch. This is where you begin to experience the auras of people other than yourself.

Find a partner willing to shake auras, not just hands. Explore, then turn to the Q&A.

1. Sit or stand facing each other.

2. One partner's right hand moves towards the other partner's right hand, and vice versa. Both hands should be in sensor position. Do an aura bounce together.

3. Notice how this shared bounce differs from doing it all by yourself. Is the energy farther out or closer? Alternate bouncing alone, then with your partner.

4. Repeat Steps #2 and 3, but substitute an aura rub for aura bounce. Here comes your chance to experience the quality of energy from your partner. Does it differ in temperature, texture, color? Experiment.

5. Repeat all of the above, but this time you and your partner can use the hand that wasn't being used before.

6. Last time around, both you and your partner should use your *primary sensor hand*. What's that? Everyone has one hand that picks up energy a little better than the other, whereas the other hand is better at sending out energy.

   The best technique I've found for sorting this out comes from Reiki Master Beth Gray.

   Clasp your hands together so your fingers interlace. The hand with the thumb on top is your *energy transmitter hand*. The other is your primary sensor hand.

7. To broaden your experience of auric touch even more, go on to repeat the aura handshake with as many people as possible.

Aura Handshake

Q. **That was fantastic. Can everyone have an experience like this?**

A. Yes, through at least one of the senses. Practice will make that subtle sense stronger and help you to clear other subtle senses, too.

Q. **Frankly, I still don't feel much. Am I hopeless?**

A. "Much" implies that you felt something. What did you notice last time you did the handshake?

Q. There were some little currents, like waves, but no big deal. Aren't auras supposed to be, you know, more significant?

A. And you were expecting something significant, right?

Q. Right. I want to see colors, something that means something.

A. The reason you don't feel much yet is that you are placing conditions on your perception. Let go of your Myth about Auras and let yourself experience according to your gifts. It's okay, really. If you simply let yourself perceive now and, later, use your inner dictionary, your aura readings will be full of meaning.

Q. But little currents and waves don't mean diddly!

A. If you despise them, they won't. Give them a chance, even if the perception comes in a way you didn't expect. That's what I mean when I say that the experience of reading auras is *new*.

Q. I'm having the opposite problem from his. Doing the handshakes, I felt so much, it was overwhelming. What if you get scared because you really do feel something?

A. First, realize that you can always use the techniques described later for unwelcome perception. Second, congratulate yourself for being so sensitive. Third, now that you know what's going on, prepare to have the rest of your life become a lot easier.

Q. Huh?

A. If you're having intense experiences already, that shows you are intuitively supersensitive. I'll bet you react intensely in other situations too, not just aura reading class. By training yourself to use your perception consciously and voluntarily, you'll be able to lighten up the rest of the time.

Q. What we're doing with the handshakes reminds me of Healing Touch. How is it different?

A. First, let's define it. Not everyone knows about Healing Touch. It's a form of aura reading and energy healing that develops subtle perception, especially clairsentience. The Colorado Center for Healing Touch, in Lakewood, Colorado, standardizes this method. Its books and classes are the best I've seen in terms of teaching subtle perception techniques in a way that encourages self-authority. Healing Touch uses the kind of perception you have developed through the techniques of aura bounce, rub, and handshake.

Q. So what's the difference?

A. Compared to Aura Reading Through All Your Senses, Healing Touch is more specialized. It has a specific purpose, healing. My multi-sense approach will help you develop all the spiritual gifts linked to your subtle senses, whether or not your gifts involve healing.

Q. What if you do want to be a healer?

A. Becoming certified in a technique like Healing Touch requires that you look for specific bits of information, for which you are taught specific interpretations and instructions. Here you aim for open-ended discovery.

Later on, as you read your inner dictionary, you will learn that there is a significance to everything you discover on your own. Now let's say that you have talent as a healer. You may discover a kind of healing not covered by Healing Touch. If all you studied was Healing Touch, you might never find your special contribution to healing.

Q. Is there a conflict between your system of aura reading and Healing Touch or other techniques?

A. Aura Reading Through All Your Senses is perfectly compatible with studying systems of healing, like Healing Touch, Therapeutic Touch, and Shiatsu, to name a few. Of course, you shouldn't hang out your shingle for professional work without technical study and formal credentials.

Still, I recommend that you explore my system as early in your study as possible because it makes you aware of your unique perceptions. Afterwards, you'll have a deeper experience with any system you study.

And remember, there are plenty of reasons aside from healing to explore aura reading, like shopping smarter, enjoying sex more, raising your consciousness for a spiritual high. You shouldn't have to go for years of formal certification training just because you want to read auras.

Telephone Awareness

Did you ever realize how much you have in common with your telephone? Talking and listening are separate. You may even hold the receiver differently when you listen versus when you talk. Communication means alternating the two. At least it should!

Whenever you have a conversation, you exchange energy. Quite apart from who is speaking, one person takes on the role of receiver while the other transmits. Sometimes people switch roles energetically. Surprisingly often they don't.

The point of the following telephone awareness technique is for you to become aware of those energy give-and-takes. Step #2 is included for contrast, helping you sort out the difference between noticing subtle psychological energy, as shown in nonverbal communication, and reading the subtler energy exchanges that involve auras. (More about these different levels will be discussed in the Q&A.)

Telephone Awareness Technique

1. Stand opposite your partner. Adjust your physical distance from each qther until both of you feel comfortable with it.

2. Shake hands—the regular physical nonaura way. Then partners return hands to their sides. Inwardly notice who takes the lead. (What you're observing here is the level of nonverbal communication, informative and fascinating but *not* aura reading.)

3. Do a slow-motion aura handshake: bounce and then rub. Pause in a rub position. Pay attention to who gives energy, who receives. How does each part feel to you? (Now you're exploring the level of aura reading.)

4. Repeat the previous steps with several different partners. What happens?

Telephone Awareness

Q. **When people are together do they always exchange energy?**

A. Yes, and not just people with people. For fun, use telephone awareness on yourself with animals or plants.

Q. **I found that I was the one who transmitted to my partner. Let me tell you, the sensation was very familiar. On reflection, I'm the one who does most of the transmitting to my friends. And it does leave me feeling drained. Are some people energy takers?**

A. You bet.

Q. **What if I want to receive more often? How can I change the pattern?**

A. Advice columnist Ann Landers often writes, "Nobody can take advantage of you without your permission." That's true of auric energy, too. If you can realize you're being taken advantage of aurically, you can change the pattern.

So pay attention to your energy exchanges. No matter whom you're with, you don't have to transmit energy unless you want to. It can help to set an inner intention: "Stop sending him energy." Then keep your awareness inside, using the centering technique described later.

On a practical level you can experiment with different behaviors, different relationships.

Q. In *The Celestine Prophecy* James Redfield wrote about control dramas, addictions, and people stealing energy from each other. It seemed kind of depressing. Am I going to find this all the time with your telephone awareness?

A. Not necessarily. I think Redfield made a valuable contribution by alerting us to the importance of energy dynamics. Sometimes you'll find control dramas but other times you'll find hidden information that is highly positive. The more fascinated you are by watching people, the more you'll enjoy adding the new level of telephone awareness.

Q. New level? What are the old levels?

A. Level #1 means noticing what happens in physical reality. Who says what? Who does what?

Q. Okay. The first level is the obvious factual stuff.

A. Level #2 involves psychological interpretation. Do you remember when you first became consciously aware of nonverbal communication? You learned to read facial expression and body language, tone of voice. Experts on nonverbal communication point out even more subtle aspects that are rarely conscious–kinesics, proxemics, microexpressions. However much you learn to notice, all behaviors reveal a deeper emotional truth than mere words.

Q. Is that aura reading, then?

A. No. But it gets tricky. Nonverbal communication is the psychological study of emotional energy. But sometimes people bring to it the subtle senses of emotional touch and emotional empathy. Then they supplement psychological study with aura reading. The previous technique for Telephone Awareness will help you sort out the difference between Levels #2 and 3.

Q. What's next?

A. Level #3 is awareness of the subtle spiritual energy that exists independently of emotional behavior.

Q. Please give an example of all three levels.

A. Let's say you're watching a longtime married couple have a conversation at the mall.

1. Obvious Reality

The couple is sitting on a bench. Their words seem polite but tense.

2. Nonverbal Communication

Body language shows that this is not a happy relationship. The woman leans towards the man in a domineering way. He squirms and fidgets. Nonverbally, they appear to have an entrenched pattern where the wife pushes the husband around. On this level, the woman is stealing energy from the man.

3. Aura Reading

You walk past the couple, just inches away from their bodies, to tap into their auras. With your primary sensor hand (or using visual techniques that come later), you pick up what is happening with their auras. Surprise! You learn that the woman is pouring huge amounts of a rather gentle, loving energy into the man.

A. **So there's actually something in it for the husband, putting up with a wife who's a rotten conversationalist and a bully!**

A. Now you know. Despite superficial problems, the people in this example share a deep connectedness, including a very positive energy transfer. Auras explain a lot.

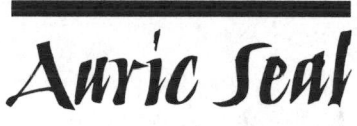

Auric Seal

To complete your introduction to touching auras, you must learn about your ethical responsibility. I know, because my ethical responsibility is to tell you about it.

After you've touched anyone's aura directly for more than a minute or two, you may well have made a significant change. Perhaps you have rearranged part of an auric layer. Perhaps you have brought in some extra spiritual energy. Perhaps you have inadvertently taken some. In any case, you need not know precisely what you have done in order to seal off the aura. In every case the technique I call "auric seal" will protect and strengthen a person's energy field.

Why bother to seal an aura? Think about your own need for personal space, personal boundaries. Have you ever been stuck in a crowded bus? Even if nobody bumps against you, afterwards you feel jostled. That's not "just" your imagination. Your fellow bus riders have unwittingly invaded your aura and dumped in their stuff. When you explore someone else's aura at length, you change it. So seal it back up afterwards.

How To Seal an Aura

1. Sit opposite a partner. One person at a time transmits the auric seal while the other receives it. Let's call the person who receives "your client." Here is what to do when it's your turn to work on your client:

2. Place your hands a few inches above where you have been touching your client's aura with any of the previous techniques. Use sensor position, both hands parallel. Your palms should face the person whose aura you want to seal.

3. Starting from the top of the head, slowly move your hands all the way to your client's feet. Then drop your hands, raise them back to starting position, and repeat the downward motion twice, for a total of three passes. This will complete the auric seal.

4. Pay attention to your experience while doing this. Afterwards ask your client for feedback.

Auric Seal

Q. **So now I'm waving my hands in the air. Isn't this getting kind of weird?**

A. It won't seem so weird once you have developed the skill to feel or see the aura in that "air." Before then, ask your client for a reaction. Did yours say anything?

Q. He liked it, I must admit. He said it felt like I was wrapping him up in a coat of energy.

Q. **Can you do an auric seal on yourself?**

A. Sure. Hold your hands in sensor position with palms inward, then move them from your head downwards as far as you can reach. The process is essentially the same whether you do it on yourself or somebody else.

Q. **Then why did you have us start doing it on somebody else?**

A. With another person's energy there is more contrast, making results more noticeable.

Q. **Could I use the auric seal on myself after getting my energy smushed in a crowd?**

A. That's a great idea. But you might want to take one precaution. Wait until you're alone. Otherwise the folks who don't see auras yet will wonder about you. Once I made quite an impression, checking out my aura from the head down by patting the air in front of me. By the time I got to the lower portions, I happened to walk right past a group of construction workers. They were entertained, to put it mildly.

Q. **Why do you stroke auras from the top down, rather than the bottom up?**

A. Since human energy flows top to bottom, it feels better to go with the flow. It's like stroking a cat's fur in the right direction.

Q. **What if I try stroking in the opposite direction?**

A. The more sensitive you are, the less you'll like how it rumples your energy. If you want to experiment, go ahead. But finish by sealing your aura in the top-down direction.

Q. **What happens when the position of your hands is too far out or too close?**

A. If your hands move out farther than three feet or so, your client probably won't be able to notice the soothing effect of the auric seal. When hands get closer than 12 inches, you're no longer doing auric seal, you're giving auric massage.

Auric Massage

It's arguably the easiest and most soothing massage in the world. Another benefit of auric massage is that it helps the giver refine clairsentient perception.

Instructions follow to massage yourself and to massage a client. Choose whichever you prefer.

Self-Massage

1. Sit comfortably in a chair.

2. With hands in sensor position, make parallel strokes from head to knees. Come as close as a couple of inches. Avoid physical touching, though. It's distracting. Experiment with the distance until you find what feels best to you. Regarding length of stroke, don't outline the body in one slow, sweeping motion, as with the auric seal. Instead use short strokes and overlap them, as if you were using a broom to sweep dust from the floor.

3. After you go from head to knees, use your right hand to brush the aura over your left arm, moving from shoulder to fingertips. Switch hands to massage the other arm.

4. If you like, also bend over to massage the aura from the top of your legs to your feet.

5. Important: After the massage, close off your aura with the auric seal from head to feet.

Client Massage

Choose your clients with care. Remember that you may be held responsible for the effects of your massage, even as a volunteer who is experimenting on a friend. Check with an attorney if you have any questions.

Also, experts at Healing Touch recommend short sessions for children and the elderly. They warn never to do energy work on someone who might be prone to a stroke. To be on the safe side, follow these restrictions for auric massage as well.

1. Ask your client to lie down on his back.

2. Use both hands to make parallel strokes from head to toes. Be sure to ask for feedback at the start of the massage to make sure your hands are at the distance your client finds most comfortable.

   During the massage, switch on telephone awareness from time to time. Are you giving energy or receiving it?

3. Have your client roll over onto his front. Massage the aura over his back, from head to heels.

4. Close with an auric seal.

5. When the massage is complete, ask your client what he noticed. It's amazing how something so easy could be so relaxing.

Auric Massage

Q. **When I played client, I felt much more than with any of the other aura touching exercises so far. Why?**

A. Maybe it's because you were relaxed, not expecting. Subtle perception is forced out by trying hard. Dr. Bill Bauman, Founder of the World Peace Institute and the smartest energy mover I've known yet, jokes about how he switches on his highest awareness by purposely "going brain dead."

Q. **My favorite part of the self-massage happened when I used my right hand—alone—over my left arm. Would there be any harm in doing a massage with just one hand?**

A. Not at all. Remember what you learned with the aura handshake? Each hand in sensor position has a specialty. One hand is a bit better at receiving, one better at giving. Primary sensor hand is the hand you've already identified as the hand that receives better. Your other hand is a built-in subtle laser blaster, your *energy transmitter hand*.

Because our emphasis in this book is on reading energy, rather than sending it, I'll be calling your energy transmitter hand by a different name: your *alternate sensor hand*.

Q. **When should I use my primary sensor hand alone?**

A. Use it alone to emphasize receiving information from an aura.

Q. **How would I make use of both hands for subtle massage?**

A. To give the massage, mostly you are sending out energy, so two hands will be more efficient than one. But, while massaging, sometimes you will feel that you are starting to receive information or energy. To follow up, take away your alternate sensor hand long enough to sort out the information available. Afterwards return your alternate sensor hand and resume moving both hands together.

Q. **Now that you mention it, when I was massaging over Jake's left leg I had a crazy idea. I thought it seemed tired. Could that be an example of receiving information?**

A. You bet. [It turned out that Jake was feeling pain from a sports injury that had been acting up recently.]

Q. **When giving this kind of massage, does it make any difference whether your client has clothes on or not?**

A. It might to your client! To the masseur, clothes shouldn't make any difference. Regardless of clothing, it wouldn't hurt to use *auric massage oil*.

Q. Auric massage oil?

A. Rub your hands back and forth. This intensifies the flow of energy from your hands. You can use this trick at any point during the massage or whenever you read auras with your hands, as with the aura bounce or rub or seal.

Q. How long should an auric massage last?

A. Good question. The auric level is far more powerful than the physical. A little bit goes a long way: 15 minutes on your client's aura could equal a 60-minute Swedish massage. Don't overdo!

Q. Much as I enjoyed doing my massage this time, knowing me, I'm sure to get bored using just one kind of stroke. Any suggestions?

A. Once you start moving your hands around in different directions, you're rearranging an aura. The effects could be dramatic, good or bad. So if you plan to get into this, I'd recommend that you prepare yourself with professional training.

Q. Auric massage feels great to me. I just wish I could see what I'm doing.

A. Maybe you are ready to do just that.

Mirror, Mirror on the Soul

Remember the shock of hearing your own voice on tape for the first time? How about seeing yourself on video? It's common to feel self-conscious, even to blow your seeming "faults" out of proportion. Seeing your energy field is a lot more pleasant.

Maybe you will start with a tantalizing glimpse of life energy (the level of aura closest to your body). Maybe you'll see a more abstract part of your aura that shows your individuality as soul (a level farther from your body). Maybe you will see one of a number of levels in between.

But no matter which level you see, and no matter how clearly, you can relax. Auras are made of light ... and for the most part, sweetness. This self-seeing technique is the first of three designed to develop your clairvoyance. Before you begin each one, read though the instructions completely. For best results the first time you try it, ask a partner to read each step aloud (afterwards you can switch roles), or prepare by tape recording the instructions, starting with Step #3. Leave three minutes of silence after Step #3, five after Step #4.

Mirror Technique

1. Prepare your environment. Find a good bathroom—or any room with a big mirror where you can have ten minutes uninterrupted. If you wear glasses or contact lenses, take them off. Perfect eyesight is not a requirement for this process. Relaxed eyesight is.

While getting ready, bring a recording device within reach. Choose a pen and paper, cassette tape recorder, or a friend with a ready ear.

2. Position yourself close enough to the mirror to see your reflection comfortably. Soften the lighting for greatest comfort. No dimmer switch? How about a night light? Or try turning off the bathroom light and leaving the door ajar. (If you still can't adjust the lighting, don't worry about it.)

3. Palm your eyes: Close them. Hold your right palm over your right eye, fingertips touching your forehead. Palm your left eye in a similar manner. Breathe slowly and deeply for a few minutes. As you relax, you will begin to see a velvety blackness. Listen for a sound of deep silence.

4. When you are ready, open your eyes and gaze towards your reflection. "Gaze towards" means the opposite of staring—look in a casual, not-minding way. Aim your eyes towards the general vicinity of your head. See whatever you see, without trying for anything specific. Continue as long as desired.

5. To signal that the session is over, blink a few times. Put on your glasses or contacts, as appropriate. Return to normal focused vision.

6. Record what you saw in the mirror. Even if you don't feel completely sure of yourself, throw some words out. Regardless of how you express your discoveries, the process of recording is valuable in itself; it sets up coordination between your languaging ability and subtle perception.

Mirror Technique

Q. **Amazing! Soon as I opened my eyes, I saw a flash of light 'round my head, about six inches thick. Then it went away. The room was pretty dark otherwise. It must have been my aura, but it didn't look the way I expected, and it had no color. Why not? I thought auras came in color.**

A. Not for every one. Be grateful for *your* experience. Learn from *your* experience. It's the truest teacher you'll ever find.

Q. **The thing I saw—if it was an aura—was small and close to my shoulders and head. It was silvery. What does that mean?**

A. You did see your aura. The meaning will be found in the next section, "Your Inner Dictionary."

Q. How about the blob of violet light I saw?

Q. Why did I see a whole lot of yellow on the left side of my head but nowhere else?

Q. What do you make of flickering lights?

A. Stay tuned for "Your Inner Dictionary."

Q. **How come no two of us saw the same thing, yet you call it all auras?**

A. Important question! There are many levels of aura to see. Each of you has a level that you gravitate towards, the level that links to your spiritual work. You might meet someone else on your wavelength who sees the same sort of thing, but I wouldn't waste my time waiting for that external validation. What matters most is your inner experience—and the extent to which you use your personal dictionary to find a rich interpretation.

Q. **At least I'm sure of what I saw. It was an afterimage. I am wearing an orange sweatshirt. The light around my shoulders was blue.**

A. That could have been an afterimage. They come in colors complementary to what you've just been looking at. (Other complementary combinations are purple and yellow, green and red.)

But unless a flashbulb went off as you looked at yourself, what you saw was probably your aura, not an afterimage.

Q. How can I know for sure?

A. Give seeing a real chance. Use the mirror technique regularly for a couple of weeks. Do it with an attitude of innocence, no expectations. Your slogan might be, "Here goes nothing." After these two weeks, you'll probably have started seeing, but if not, use your other senses instead and let the visual part of aura reading sneak up on you.

Q. Instead of seeing an aura, I gave myself a headache. Is this common?

A. If you try hard, definitely. Hard work can make a person extremely successful at things in physical reality, but auras are a subtle reality. Trying won't help. It hinders. And it can even hurt, as you now know.

Next time you use this technique, don't strain to see. Avoid staring or blinking. Forget about any way of using your eyes to focus hard. If anything, allow your eyes to go *out* of focus. Your celestial sight will develop naturally once you give it a chance, so relax and enjoy yourself.

Auric sight usually starts as peripheral vision, unexpected little flashes you see out of the corner of your eye.

My other recommendation is that you reread the section in Chapter Two on "The Myth About Auras." Touching auras didn't give you a headache because you didn't think it was as big a deal as seeing. Well, seeing isn't such a big deal either!

Q. What I saw might have been a big deal. My face misted over until another face appeared superimposed over it. What on earth was that?

A. Probably it was an image of yourself in a past life. Before explaining further, here's an important clarification for everyone who does NOT believe in past lives.

Aura reading does not involve a belief system, other than the belief that reading auras is possible. If you don't believe in past lives—and many aura readers don't—skip ahead to the next topic.

Q. Okay, about that past life image, why was it there?

A. Your spiritual self wanted you to connect up with something about that life. As always, your inner dictionary will provide the best information.

Q. Is there any way I can use a mirror to see my past lives on purpose?

A. Yes, and it ought to be cheaper than buying a crystal ball! While your eyes are closed (Step #3), put in a simple request like this: "Higher Self (for definition, see Glossary), please show me the version of myself in a past life that would be most helpful for me to see at this time... or something better." Then go ahead with the rest of the process. If it's in your best interest to see yourself in a past life, you will.

Synesthesia Surprises

Now that you have had the chance to explore techniques for sight as well as touch, let's pause to acknowledge something important but subtle that you may have experienced along the way.

Use of one subtle sense can wake up other subtle senses. Synesthesia makes this possible.

For instance:

- When Carlo practiced the aura handshake he saw light come out of his partner's hand. It blended with the light from his own. "Wow!" he said. "When I touch, I see."

- Before Rhonda's teacher could finish giving the instructions for the mirror technique, Rhonda interrupted, "I'm seeing them already. Started while you were talking!" In addition to seeing the teacher's aura, emotional touch added to Rhonda's insights.

- Clairaudience came, more than the colors Margaret expected, when she did the mirror technique. Clairaudience didn't come automatically, though. Here's what happened.

Margaret seemed to notice nothing visually when she looked in the space over her shoulders and around her head. But she had a bright idea. She framed a question this way:

"What information about auras is available to me from what I'm looking at?"

Immediately she began to *hear* information. It happened to be about health, which turned out to be one of her main specialties as an aura reader.

This process has continued for Margaret. When she looks for an aura, she picks up information through questioning, then hearing. That's her formula for a way in.

- Psychic knowing surprised Tim. In the midst of aura massage he felt that he knew many specific things about his client's past. Verified by the client, to Tim's amazement, all the psychic knowing turned out to be true. As he developed aura reading skills, Tim found that subtle touch became a consistent trigger for psychic knowing and other subtle senses.

- Betsy wasn't used to thinking of herself in connection with either psychic knowing or being gustatorily gifted. But then she had her synesthesia surprise. It came while she practiced telephone awareness between herself and all the plants and flowers in the room. Dried flowers, displayed in a vase, had an aura that was small in size but ... strong with scent. Betsy clearly experienced how the yellow chrysanthemums had smelled in full bloom.

Synesthesia experiences like these are celestial bonuses, extra perceptions you didn't even try to have. Of course it would be desirable to experience them on a regular basis. Trying harder won't do it. But you can choose to stay open and receptive. Techniques to make this happen can be as simple as asking a question. Next time you are touching or seeing an aura, ask questions that relate to other subtle senses:

- What fragrance would be part of this experience?
- Could my emotional touch give me more information? What?

- Which knowledge would enable me to be of greatest service to the person whose aura I'm reading?

Something else you can do concerns your reaction to experiences like this. "Crazy," Kim said. "I wonder if I'm losing my mind." Heather called it "scary."

"Unsettling" was Fletcher's reaction. Negative labels like these will not serve your development as an aura reader. Admittedly aura reading knocks down some of the boundary walls of everyday knowledge. Synesthesia knocks them down even flatter. Eventually these subtle experiences can move you into a different state of consciousness, where the rigid old boundaries hardly remain at all. But what's so bad about that?

Higher States of Consciousness

Waking, sleeping, dreaming—these are the familiar states of consciousness. But higher states are possible, even desirable. Here's an overview.

1. Transcendental Consciousness

This beginner's state of spiritual enlightenment occurs when you slip into an inner calmness or silence. Awake inside but physically relaxed, you experience more to life than usual.

> **Awareness of the transcendent often begins
> when you are alone.**

Meditation or prayer can do it. So can a walk in the country, quiet listening to music, a trip to the art museum. Have you ever woken up in the middle of the night to find yourself buzzing with an expanded awareness? Don't fear such experiences. Welcome them.

2. Cosmic Consciousness

Repeated experience of the transcendent leads to a new state of consciousness where you, personally, identify with inner silence. Those who are religiously minded could call it the presence of God. In cosmic consciousness, you draw your personal identity from this spiritual energy. Though you may introduce yourself by name, affiliate yourself with a race, define yourself through family, country, or job, nevertheless you know as a peaceful certainty that you are more than this.

> **In truth you are an energy presence
> that happens to live in your body.**

A specific Aha! experience can come from deep inside when you recognize this to be true. Once and for all, you know who you are. This realization is spiritual enlightenment. Metaphysically it's a point of no return. Afterwards you may, temporarily, become caught up in the drama of everyday life. But when you pause to recollect who you truly are, the big Self is there, in all its serenity and joy.

3. Celestial Consciousness

Another aspect of higher consciousness is to pay attention to the presence of God outside yourself. Ta da—here comes the blue jeans analogy of higher states of awareness. For years you may work on looking good in your jeans: exercise, diet, endless shopping for the most flattering style. Another approach is to say, "Okay, I'm going to accept the body and clothes I have now." Then you can stop fixing, start appreciating.

That's like the shift from cosmic consciousness to celestial consciousness. After working hard to find the presence of spirit within, you have realized the Self. So now you're ready to seek God's presence in your outer life.

Many people get stuck for years in this search due to one simple mistake. Genuine spiritual experience is not the same as having ideas or feelings about being spiritual. For instance, a sermon in church may be inspiring; the happy expression on a fellow worshipper may be contagious; blessings may be counted and praise given. Well and good, but none of this is necessarily celestial consciousness.

More than a mood, discovering a higher state of consciousness involves a benign kind of inner earthquake that shakes you and wakes you up. Back at the blue jeans analogy, consider looking for labels. The manufacturer of your favorite brand sews a label into every pair. It may take a bit of looking to find that label, but you always can.

Where would you look for God's "label" in a person, a gemstone, a flower, a pet? You read it in the subtle, celestial perception of an aura. You make the choice to shift your attention, find your way in, and there you are.

Blue, fizzy, tender, perfect, surprisingly fresh—whatever the experience, it changes you. One particular celestial perception may happen once and never again. Still, a pattern of recognition develops. You learn to find the label that identifies The Celestial Manufacturing Company Unlimited.

For instance, I'll never forget the shock the first time I made conscious contact with angels. Deep in meditation, I saw and felt the beauty of a golden honeycomb. Inside it were many exquisite little babies (cherubs is the name for this kind of angel, I later found out). The angels drew closer and closer.

Inwardly I was in a state of Wow: "This is so beautiful. This is so incredibly beautiful. This is so beautiful, it's celestial."

Suddenly I realized those babies weren't just like angels, they were angels. Immediately they vanished. I had become too excited, in mind and body, to maintain the perception. Celestial consciousness sneaks up on you like that, in starts and flashes.

Will you react, as I did, by jumping like a startled deer? Maybe you will feel your hair stand on end or a shiver go through you like lightning. Perhaps time will stand still and, afterwards, for hours or days, time will soften to an exquisite tenderness. Ice cold tears of gratitude or longing may fall, slowly, from your eyes. Whatever your experiences, don't expect to ever grow entirely used to them. Still, eventually, familiarity can help you handle celestial perception with a more serene joyous acceptance.

Ask for It

Millions of Americans have had mystical experiences. Even a few seconds' worth changes your whole life. Some of my students have reported these breakthrough glimpses of celestial perception:

- Checking her aura, Renata experienced herself as a baby, cradled by God.
- Marya, a devout Christian, felt healing energy pour out of her hands as she did auric massage.
- Ed found himself in the physical presence of the Buddha.

Celestial perception could be called the experience of heaven on earth. But you can take an active role while waiting for this kind of heaven. You can choose to shift your consciousness. If you want to meet God you don't have to play hard to get. Go ahead, make a date.

Pray to the personal aspect of God who means the most to you, such as Jesus, Mary, Mohammed, or Krishna. Don't just ask for a sign. Ask for a sight or a sound, direct experience in terms of your very human subtle senses.

What if you don't feel ready? Ask to be made ready.

Can you dictate exactly when and how God will give you a clear experience of what you hold most sacred? No, but you can ask for the what. And once you've asked, why not ready yourself by becoming familiar with the celestial realms through aura reading?

Already you may have noticed. Daily practice of aura reading techniques does change your perception. When you remember to look deeper, colors become more beautiful. Music transports you nearer to the level of the composer's inspiration. Fragrances can send you into a state of bliss. Even sex could become more enjoyable.

In any situation, you can ask to read auras. Make your inner request. Use whatever subtle senses come most easily. Ask for information. Then let go. Be silent long enough to receive what you have asked for.

If your motivation is spiritual service, you will accelerate the development of celestial consciousness. Synesthesia will bring you wonders.

Artists, musicians, and poets have dedicated their lives to communicating their celestial perception. For example, Gerard Manley Hopkins was a Christian mystic whose poetry was exceptionally rich in synesthesia. A typical poem begins like this:

The world is charged with the grandeur of God.
It will flame out, like shining from shook foil;

As you develop celestial consciousness, you will find that the presence of God intensifies. You will be given as much of the experience as you can accept. Therefore, your rate of development of celestial consciousness is linked to your answer to this question: Just how much joy, beauty, and wonder can you handle?

Gratitude shows you can handle more. Fear shows you don't feel ready. Whatever your degree of inner readiness, choose your speech accordingly. To label a new experience "weird" or "scary" is to screech on the brakes.

It's understandable when someone fears a new state of consciousness. Making friends with others who also experience higher consciousness, such as other aura readers, can be reassuring.

What a shame that, with all that the media bring us daily, they have not yet educated the world very well about higher states of consciousness. Instead television, in particular, has filled the minds of Americans with images of sickness. People who have character disorders or deep pathology, even those who are psychotic, flaunt their craziness on talk shows. Stories of criminals, danger, and violence trigger everyone's fear of the unknown.

But higher states of consciousness are not of this order. If you function from a baseline of emotional stability; if you can hold a job (though you need not, necessarily, have one that pays as much as you'd like); if you don't take drugs or drink excessively; if you would *not* be a candidate for crazy talk show guest; consider yourself normal. Whatever that is! In the strange world where we live, normal does not always feel terribly normal.

And if you are basically normal, you have every right to welcome experiences of higher states of consciousness. Don't fear them, trivialize them, or make fun of them. If you welcome them, glimpses of celestial consciousness can become your everyday reality. As a result you'll enjoy greater happiness within, give more kindness to others, lead a more fulfilling life all around.

The Inner Side of Aura Reading

In the spiritual terms we've been considering, aura reading represents a meeting point between developing celestial consciousness from deep inside and turning your attention out through your senses. Fittingly, a full aura reading has two parts, outside and inside.

Part One you have now set in motion: *gathering* subtle sense data from the outside through techniques for clairsentience and clairvoyance. Part Two involves a contemplative approach, seeking information from the inside for *interpreting* subtle sense data.

Interpretation is indispensable.
Otherwise you will not value your perceptions.
Not only will you miss out.
So will the people who could have been helped
by your wisdom.

Here's the formula that will empower you:

Subtle perception + interpretation = aura reading

To access information about subtle perception you need to consult a reference book, but which one?

Your Best Reference Book

Red auras mean anger. No, red auras mean lust. No, red auras mean jealousy.

Depends on whose book you read. Let's face it, if it were possible for any expert to write the definitive aura encyclopedia, it would long since have become a standard reference book for every spiritual seeker. Remember, though, auras are about spiritual truth, not physical reality. By definition, there can be no such thing as a universal dictionary for every aura reader.

Though some expert aura readers have tried to write definitive books, they contradict each other. That should tell you something.

Besides, which do you want to do, spend your time comparing what other people perceive or reading auras yourself?

**Spiritual projects are do-it-yourself,
much as we might sometimes wish it were otherwise.
Aura reading is no exception.**

For experience of celestial perception, who has to do the work? Sure the grace of God helps, but you know the old saying, Heaven helps those who help themselves.

Now that it's time to look for meaning, the same question comes up: Who has to do the work? Again, the answer is you—*the one who will enjoy the benefits* of doing your spiritual homework.

Spiritual Homework

Shortcuts don't necessarily work with spiritual matters. To adopt another aura reader's meanings is like looking up the answers at the back of the math book. For aura reading homework, we definitely must find our own answers. Otherwise they do us very little good.

For example, I was fascinated to read about Michael Crichton's flirtation with aura reading as recounted in his autobiographical book, *Travels*. First Crichton attended a two-week conference with Dr. Brugh Joy, revered for a particular "definitive" system of auric healing. Michael succeeded in learning this, as did other participants. They saw auras Joy's way, agreed on identical colors, the same "energy findings."

But shortly after returning home, Michael reported feeling discouraged. "The energy work was real, the meditations were real, but what good was it. . . ?"

Years later, Crichton recounted, he studied for two weeks with a famous psychic, Carolyn Conger. Her way of seeing was different but Michael mastered that, too. He excelled at seeing colors around people, as the group of students gave each other external validation. But how did Crichton use it?

"When I got home, I looked at people to see if I could still see auras. I could. It's fun to do. When the dinner parties get boring, you just look at people's auras."

Fun? Yes, but that's a pretty trivial use for a gift that could have been life transforming.

Now I'm not suggesting that we feel too sorry for Michael Crichton, given his stellar success with novels and films. Nor do I wish to criticize the two teachers with whom he studied. Both sound eminently worthy of respect. But here's the problem (based on my interpretation of Crichton's account).

Both teachers had developed and refined a specialty as an aura reader. Their mistake was to pass along their specialties, dictionary and all. External validation made Crichton and his classmates feel good. What if, instead, they had been challenged to take a slower and more vulnerable route? What if they had been asked to find their own meanings, linked directly to strengths for perception and inner spiritual mission?

It boggles the mind to imagine the results if either of Crichton's aura reading teachers had encouraged him to read his own dictionary. Instead of *Jurassic Park*, Crichton might have brought the world a novel about angelic DNA. He might have become as brilliant an aura reader as he is a writer.

To develop the full brilliance of your aura reading, you need a *personal* reference book. You need it to be written in your own language, whatever words make the deepest sense to you, because the new ideas it explains will be subtle, stretching your conscious mind.

Besides that, your dictionary had better be handy, with listings and cross-references galore. Who wants to feel like a tourist, thumbing desperately through pages of useless idioms before you find the words for "Where's the bathroom?"

Fortunately, the perfect aura dictionary is available when you do your homework with the following technique.

How to Read Your Inner Dictionary

Before you start, read through all the instructions. For best results, the first *several* times you try this technique, ask a partner to read each step as appropriate (afterwards you can switch roles), or else record the instructions on a tape recorder, leaving three-minute pauses after Steps #3 and 9.

1. Just as if you were using a physical dictionary, your first task is to figure out what you want to know. Since you must shift into a deeper consciousness during your research, write down a list of questions in advance. These questions should be specific, such as:

   - "What does it mean that, when I did the aura handshake, Melissa's aura felt spongy?"

   - "When I looked at my aura, the light around my head was spiky, like the halo on the Statue of Liberty? Where's the message in that?"

   - "With the aura rub, the area located around my throat felt stuck. It sounded like a hacking cough. What was going on?"

2. The meditation to consult your inner dictionary will take some time. Allow 10-15 minutes.

   Prepare your environment. Find a comfortable, quiet place to sit, well ventilated, where you won't be interrupted by people, pets, pagers, or phones. Bring along a pad and pen, or an audio cassette player set to record.

Should your environment include soothing music? Since your goal is to read your dictionary at will, no matter where you are, I recommend that you not become dependent on music. Besides, you can relax without it. In the long run, silence works better.

Irrelevant thoughts may seem distracting, but you can handle them by gently focusing on your breathing. Or listen to the silence around you. Does it have a texture, a sound of its own?

3. Close your eyes. Mentally ask to be connected to your Higher Self.

   For two minutes or longer, take *vibe-raising breaths*. These involve long deep in-breaths through the nose and out-breaths through the mouth, plus the overall desire to go deeper within.

4. Mentally set an intention.

   Even the world's best computer won't run software without a command, so put together a simple sentence or two to give your mind a context. For example: "Higher Self, help me now to read and understand my inner dictionary."

   Next state your motivation. Express the highest purpose that feels true to you. A pure motivation feels good, so it raises your vibrations, lessens the pressure of self-doubt, and helps you feel worthy to accept wonderful knowledge. Examples: "My purpose is to be of service to others." "I wish to gain wisdom."

   Think your intention and motivation in words, but don't speak them aloud. Inwardness directs your awareness and keeps it moving in a subtle, deepening direction.

5. Return to your Higher Self. To do this, take three more vibe-raising breaths. Be open to feeling the silence of this inner space. Perhaps you will see a light or hear a sound. Don't try to force one. Rather, enjoy whatever is given to you to experience.

Possibly, you may have a feeling of opening up, either physically or emotionally. Move at your own speed without worrying about how fast you're going. In every case, once you set your intention, you can be sure that you are in direct alignment with your Higher Self. You are being given the clearest experience you can handle right now.

6. Mentally ask one question from your list of questions, then release it. Immediately take three vibe-raising breaths.

   Ideally, this process of releasing should be effortless, like dropping a stone into a still pond. After you let the stone go, you wait for the pond to do its thing, and it will respond with a pattern of ripples—the answer to your question.

7. Write down the first words that pop into your mind. Or, if you have a tape recorder handy, speak out your first thought. Keep your eyes closed for as much as the recording time as possible, and when you complete your answer, close your eyes. Return to your Higher Self with another vibe-raising breath.

   Now is not the time to evaluate or judge what comes to you. You'll be able to do that fruitfully at Step #11. Before then introspection would be a distraction. Anyway, *in*trospection would be superfluous. You're already in.

8. To find the answer to another item from your list of questions, repeat Steps #6 and 7. Cycle through the process of asking and answering until you go through your whole list or you feel tired—whichever comes first. (It's better not to read your inner dictionary when fatigued, strained, or upset. Your readings will not be accurate.)

9. Conclude your session of dictionary reading. Mentally express a few words of gratitude to your Higher Self. It can be as simple as "Thank you." Then take seven *grounding breaths.*

For each grounding breath, exhale by puffing the air out hard enough to make a blowing sound. Inhale, taking a shallow breath through the mouth and nose together. Combined with your intent to connect with the physical environment around you, grounding breaths will be an effective way to bring your awareness back to physical reality.

10. Take three minutes for transition time before opening your eyes.

    This time is your investment to prevent physiological roughness (i.e., grumpiness) caused by moving too fast from a higher vibrational state back to regular functioning. Stretch. Wiggle your toes. Open eyes slowly.

11. Go over the answers you have recorded. Now is the appropriate time to evaluate your information. And to appreciate the wisdom you have found.

Inner Dictionary

Q. Why the emphasis on starting the dictionary reading slowly and coming out slowly?

A. The deeper the state from which you ask your questions, the deeper your answers. Ideally you're in an altered state and it takes time to reach it. Mind and body are connected, so allow for a period of physical transition.

Q. What does "Higher Self" mean?

A. It's a way of referring to your Higher Power. Alternatively you could call on God, a spiritual master, or the angels who work with your energy.

> **You know which high-vibrational, loving intelligence
> you feel most comfortable asking for inner knowledge.
> Substitute your preferred language
> for my use of "Higher Self."**

Q. Why get into an altered state at all? Don't all the answers ultimately come from you?

A. Excellent question. If you answer in the middle of everyday conscious activity, your answer will come from your everyday conscious mind. If you take just one minute to enter your meditation, your answers will be relatively glib, coming from shallow reaches of your subconscious. But a deep meditation enables your answers to come from the part of you that is not distracted by daily concerns.

Q. Since, as you say, glib isn't good, why go for the first answer that pops up?

A. Now you're coming from an altered state which is anything but superficial or glib. Since you've taken precautions to move into this state of inner knowing, your first answer will be fresh and full of wisdom. But the longer you mull answers over, the more likely they will be distorted by doubts or habitual patterns of conscious thinking.

Q. Is that why we're supposed to write down our answers or tape record them?

A. Exactly. Tear them apart, if you must, after you open your eyes. Otherwise, do you really want to do a meditation where you ask for inner guidance, then spend most of your time picking it apart? Usually you'll be pleasantly surprised with the wisdom from your inner dictionary.

Q. Those nasty doubts! Any other tips on getting rid of them?

A. Just one:

> **Starting now, eliminate from your vocabulary the expression, "I don't know." This programs your subconscious mind into a state of conflict because the deepest part of you really *does* know.**

Q. I don't know if this is a doubt or just a lack of belief, but...

A. —Oops, you don't know? Start again, please.

Q. Okay, my intention was to connect with my guardian angels and, frankly, I think they stood me up.

A. Why?

Q. My mind was quiet. No bells. No whistles. Nary a wing.

A. Listen, don't fire your angels. Why should they need props? Trust that they were there for you as consciousness, merged with your own.

Q. So, what were *your* answers to the three questions you gave as examples?

A. I'll tell you but remember, these are my answers, expressed in my personal language:

Q. "What does it mean that, when I did the aura handshake, Melissa's aura felt spongy ?"

A. Her awareness is very porous. On the plus side, she is extremely receptive to learning from other people. On the minus side, she has trouble setting personal boundaries and knowing her own mind. Aura reading can help her solve these problems.

Q. "When I looked at my aura, the light around my head was spiky, like the halo on the Statue of Liberty? Where's the message in that?"

A. You saw the symbol of a new energy, a spiritual quality that represents a new level of freedom. Spiritually, your Higher Self is showing you a monument, all right. It's your personal Statue of Liberty.

Q. **"With the aura rub, the area around my throat felt stuck. It sounded like a hacking cough. What was going on?"**

A. This represents a long-term sadness about communication. It's a feeling that others won't listen when you talk, so why bother? Yet desire to communicate continues, along with the hope that this time your words will be heard.

Q. **What if you don't understand an answer? One time all I got was "grayish blue."**

A. That's a great start! Your next question should follow up. For instance, "What is the meaning of grayish blue?"

If, for example, according to your dictionary, one man's grayish blue aura means "hopefulness," then that's what it will mean when you see grayish blue around other people as well.

Once your inner dictionary gives you a meaning you can understand, you put in place a new item of your spiritual vocabulary.
Keep a notebook or journal, if you like, and write down each entry.

Q. **You said we could use the inner dictionary to see our past lives. How?**

A. First, do the mirror technique. Set an intention to see yourself in a past life. Say that you see an odd expression in your eyes, then a strange costume at your neckline, then (gasp!) grayish blue light around your head.

Close your eyes immediately. Consult the inner dictionary. Here are some of the questions you might ask:

- What is the meaning of the odd expression I saw in my eyes?
- What time period did my costume come from?
- Tell me more about the person who wore the costume.
- What was the significance of the grayish blue light around my head?
- What life lesson can I learn from that past incarnation?

Q. Didn't you also say we could use the inner dictionary to improve the faculty you called psychic knowing? How would that work?

A. Ask questions that pertain to psychic knowing. **The trick is to make them open ended, rather than a yes-no question.** So don't ask, "Will I ever find true love?" Ask, "Tell me about my future husband."

Q. How about surfing through your dictionary like the Internet, to move you into another space or time?

A. For this, **set up a sequence of requests and questions**, for example:

- Higher Self, please connect me energetically to my sister in Montana.
- What is going on with her health right now?
- What is the spiritual cause of this problem?
- Which part of this information would it be helpful for me to share?
- Higher Self, please disconnect me energetically from my sister.

Q. Disconnect? That's a surprise. Should you always ask for a disconnect at the end of the reading?

A. Yes. That's important. Otherwise you stay psychically connected, which can cause confusion. Aura reading, like life in general, works better when you operate from a state of clarity.

Unwelcome Perception

Empathic experience isn't all sweetness and light. What if you're haunted by images of sadness, pain, or other unwelcome perceptions? The following techniques should help.

1. Dealing with Specific Situations

After an unwelcome emotion or physical sensation sneaks up on you, eventually you will become aware of it. Make an agreement with yourself that, starting now, you will become consciously aware of these acquisitions *right away*, as soon as you take them on. This, alone, can make a big difference. The longer a sensation clings to you, the harder it is to shake. So ask your Higher Self to signal you whenever psychic cleanup is necessary.

Once you become aware that you need to do a cleanup, speak out words like these:

Whatever does not belong to me, [say your full name here], please leave immediately.

It will, except in rare instances.

To satisfy your curiosity, you can ask for information about the real source of whatever you were feeling. Just ask your inner dictionary.

2. Choosing to Be of Service

A further option is to choose to be of service to the one whose pain you felt. You can obtain more information from your inner dictionary, then take action. Let's say that a pain leaves your right knee. You question, "Who really owns that knee pain?" The answer is, "Susan, my best friend." You can pursue this further. "Why does she have that pain?" Intuition informs you that she feels angry at her husband; she feels he is bossing her around.

If you still wish to help and assuming, too, that your inner guidance says that Susan might be receptive, you could say something like this, "My intuition has told me that you're feeling angry now. Is it true?" By opening the door to discussion, you provide an opportunity for your friend to move energy.

> **Incidentally, it's a good idea to use humility when sharing information that comes from your inner dictionary. It will be your truth, expressed in the form of your personal symbols.**

Susan's version of "husband bossing her around" might be "my supervisor at work just cut my hours."

Keep in mind, when you free yourself from being psychically tied to an unwelcome sensation, you are under no obligation, spiritually or otherwise, to volunteer for additional service. Don't burn yourself out.

3. Keeping Yourself Clear

It's really a big deal to recognize that you have a gift like emotional empathy, physical empathy, or psychic knowing. Learning to release unwelcome perception can be a breakthrough. Aside from knowing how to deal with problem situations, you now have the option of doing maintenance on a daily basis.

This maintenance takes only a minute or two, provided you know what to do. To me, it's as routine as brushing teeth.

Every morning, speak the following affirmation out loud: *"I am in control of my mind. I balance the objective and subjective sides of reality."*

These words, adapted from The Teaching of the Inner Christ, will remind you to keep your subtle insights in perspective. Overinterpreting experience is a danger for any sensitive person. The goal is to engage actively as a participant in reality, inwardly aware but not obsessed.

Once you have used this affirmation to get your day off to a good start, situations may still come up where you become caught up in unwelcome perception. Whenever you feel the need to regain psychic balance, you repeat the affirmation. The section on "Centering" in Chapter Four is an excellent follow-up.

In rare cases, despite all your efforts, unwelcome perceptions can return. Depending on the intensity, you may need to seek professional help from a spiritual counselor, psychiatrist, or other appropriate health practitioner. But in most cases, it's enough to ignore unwelcome perceptions. Don't feed them with fear or worry. Let them fade into the background, eventually disappearing entirely.

Remember, the purpose of your subtle perception is not to make you a victim. If that has been your spiritual agreement with the Universe, you are free to change it.

Often we have agreements, deep expectations, that we're not even aware of consciously. If you even suspect that you suffer in life because of a limiting agreement, you have the spiritual right to ask for a change. And often that change comes in a way that's surprisingly easy.

For instance, you might say, "I now make a new agreement with the Universe. The purpose of my subtle perception is to bring joy and personal evolution. I always have the ability to adjust the amount of perception to keep myself in balance."

Unwelcome Perception

Q. My friend George is always seeing negative forces around people, like dishonesty and anger. Isn't it sad his spiritual gift is to see only that?

A. Repeated or overwhelming negative thoughts are not a spiritual gift. They are a psychological problem. Please urge him to seek counseling from a therapist or spiritual counselor.

Q. Could empathy cause physical problems? I've been called a hypochondriac but I'm beginning to think I just have what you call physical empathy. I think I've suffered enough. I want to stop picking up pain from others. But—does this sound stupid?— I don't want to turn off my spiritual gift—if it is one.

A. The techniques just given for unwelcome perception can clear your pain without turning off your spiritual gift.

Q. But if I release unwelcome perceptions right away, I won't even remember them long enough to look them up in my inner dictionary.

A. Carry a little notebook. When you notice an unwelcome sensation, jot down what you felt and where, along with a few details about the circumstances. Then use your affirmation to clear the experience from you, personally. You'll be amazed at how much you can learn, pain free.

Q. The colors I've been seeing aren't a pain, but I do find it troubling that they come without my asking. How can I turn them off for part of the time without stopping them for all of the time?

A. When you don't want the colors, affirm: "I am in control of my mind. For now, I choose to be aware of objective reality only." When you do want the colors, say inwardly: "I call on my Higher Self to show me this person's aura."

The key to aura reading, for you, is to know that you are always in control.

Q. **When I walked into a hotel room during my last vacation, I looked in the mirror and heard: "The man who stayed here before you didn't like what he saw when he looked in the mirror."**

A. That was psychic knowing.

Q. **Okay, psychic knowing. How can I keep it from spooking me out?**

A. In the case you mentioned, I think your perception had a purpose. Did you know that people leave psychic debris after them? You can feel it in hotel rooms, offices, your local Department of Motor Vehicles.

If you're going to stay a while in a place that has bad vibes, you can psychically houseclean by burning incense or camphor, using a smudge stick, or opening a window for half an hour or longer.

Or try this method: Open a window. Burn incense. Then wave a *clean* towel around the room, including corners.

Q. **Some of my perceptions are spooky. I got a letter from my brother and started to smell tangerines out of nowhere. Without opening the envelope, I knew that he was in trouble. Sure enough, he was feeling sad about a romantic breakup. But what did that have to do with tangerines?**

A. That's a question for your inner dictionary. Really, it doesn't sound as though this knowing was deeply disturbing. It just surprised you, and this time the news happened to be bad. If you want to develop intuitively, avoid putting down your perceptions, okay?

Q. But people always joke about that sort of thing, don't they? I guess I joke to avoid coming across as stuck up. I don't want to sound like I can do something other people can't.

A. But everyone can read auras! I think you'll do everyone a favor if you treat your own readings with respect.

Every professional aura reader I've known has a wacky sense of humor, but none of them ridicule their God-given gifts. Jokes about "spooky" or "scary" perceptions promote misunderstanding. Or they can be an indirect form of bragging.

Q. Yesterday I was driving down the highway while a car accident was being cleared away. Because I'm an emotional empath, I instantly felt the strong emotions of those who had been in the crash. This didn't help anyone, and it made me feel sick. What would you have done in my place?

A. Ask: "Does this really belong to me? If not, please leave immediately." Then send a prayer in the direction of the people by the side of the road— or visualize sending them a beam of golden light.

Auravision

This technique develops your ability to see at will the auras of anyone and everyone.

With practice, seeing auras can be as simple as switching on a television.

---

1. Find a partner with whom you can share this process. For each of you, the other will be "the client." Sit across from each other, preferably each of you against a wall that is one solid color (avoid patterned wallpaper or paintings).

2. Gently direct your gaze to your client's third eye—the spot between the eyebrows. If your sight wanders away from this spot, that's okay. But if you find you have been looking elsewhere, calmly bring your eyes back.

3. Mentally set an intention to see your client's aura for your own growth of wisdom or (if applicable) to be of service.

4. Palm your eyes for a few minutes.

5. Open your eyes and gaze towards your client. Aim your eyes towards the vicinity of your client's head. Notice whatever you notice—no trying for anything specific. But for extra fun, play with any of the following variations:

   - Avoid blinking—not to the point where you cause physical discomfort but as a way of letting your eyes unfocus.

- Squint a few inches above your client's head and shoulders.
- Point your vision about four feet above your partner's head. In slow motion, let your gaze slide down the air, as if you are more interested in light and air than in the wall behind your partner. Do you see any fluctuations within the air, such as flickering, currents of air, space that looks—somehow—different? That's aura!
- Experiment with the lighting in the room. Make it bright, dim, or dark.
- Place a dark piece of fabric (navy or black) in back of your partner's head before you begin to look.

6. Take 2-3 minutes for transition time. Blink a few times. Stretch. Yawn. Return to normal, focused vision.

7. Describe to your partner what you saw.

- Avoid expressions that belittle your experience, such as "I'm not sure about this, but…" or "This wasn't very important." Any experience, no matter how subtle or vague, could be important.
- Also don't go into detail about all the things you *didn't* see. It's a waste of time.

Aura reading is new, remember? It's as if you are learning to balance on a two-wheeler for the first time. Wobbliness is a given, so don't dwell on it. Congratulate yourself for your courage in learning to ride and keep on pedaling. Or, in this case, keep on talking about your perceptions, regardless of doubts.

8. Consult your inner dictionary for further information about what you saw. Tell these interpretations to your partner and ask for feedback.

9. Give thanks for what you've been shown and for the continued development of your inner sight.

Auravision

Q. **So I saw a little light. Whoopee. What was the point?**

A. That kind of light is your way in to seeing and reading auras. Maybe it isn't the flashy kind of experience you were expecting, but it is *your* experience and could turn out to be very useful. One professional psychic I know also sees simple light, in varying amounts, when she looks at her clients' auras. Consulting her inner dictionary, she derives insights for which her clients are very grateful. Incidentally, they pay her well, too.

Q. **I did see a kind of golden light around my partner, but that's not the kind of light that people see if they can see auras.**

A. Play back what you just said! Oops. Please don't put down your experience. It is part of your spiritual gift.

Q. **Look, I can pretend to be positive as well as the next guy, but the truth is that no matter what I see, it could be my imagination. How can I be sure I'm not just making things up?**

A. You're not. But what would be the crime if you were?

Most of us were raised to believe in just one truth, objective reality. But human experience has many truths: physical, emotional, energetic, mythic, spiritual.

One of the clearest clairvoyants I know began by imagining auras on purpose. Gradually Joanna discovered that these imaginary things were real. The playfulness of pretending was what Joanna's subconscious mind needed to break through her conscious resistance. Once she acknowledged her intuitive abilities, this awesomely powerful healer stopped feeling as though she was pretending. She *knew* that she knew.

Q. **Well I know that I got some information from your auravision technique, and the process wasn't difficult. But it took a lot of psychic energy, much more than if I just used my primary sensor hand. Seeing doesn't feel like my way. Is there any reason why I should use it if feeling comes easier?**

A. No. To read an aura you only need one way in. You're wise to recognize the way that works best for you.

Q. **Seeing auras is fun for me, and not hard. I'd like to do more of it. Can you suggest a way to see auras on people other than a designated partner.**

A. Your auravision set is totally portable. Bring it wherever you can observe another person for a few minutes without attracting undue attention.

Some good places to read auras are: concerts, theaters, restaurants, work, school. Athletic events can be fascinating auric productions. And next time you go to an amusement park, wait in line for the biggest roller coaster. Watch the people who get off.

Q. **What if all I can see is the back of a head?**

A. That should work fine. Auras stick out in back as well as in front.

Q. **Any other tips for auravision in everyday situations?**

A. Even though people's auras stick out from their physical bodies, your best preparation for seeing them is to prepare to go inward, not outward. Take a few minutes to settle into a quiet, meditative state.

Libraries, theaters, and churches are places where you can physically close your eyes without seeming strange. In other places, look down at your lap or pretend to be reading. Inconspicuously take some vibe-raising breaths.

Once you feel settled, look up and read auras. Jot down questions in your notebook for later research with your inner dictionary.

Inner Sight

Subtle sight can also be approached as a form of contemplation with eyes closed. For some people it's easier when clairvoyance doesn't have to compete with regular vision.

> **People with visual disabilities can have profound inner experiences of subtle light.**

One of my students, Steve, had been blind since the age of three. Total darkness was all he saw, until he learned meditation. Then he saw a bright white light. It came, he said, every time he meditated.

Another woman I've known, Carol, combined vivid auric sight with extremely impaired vision. Fascinated by the subtle stuff, she would forget to pay attention to her physical surroundings. Stumbling over things became a way of life. Inner sight, while sitting down, might have saved her some bruises. The following method is suitable for anyone who wishes to explore clairvoyance.

Inner Clairvoyance

1. Position yourself in a room the same way as for the mirror technique or auravision. If you don't have a partner to hear your feedback, bring along equipment for writing or audiotaping.

2. Turn awareness inward by taking plenty of vibe-raising breaths. Close your eyes. Set your intention and palm your eyes until you see the blackness beneath closed eyes. Listen for any sound of silence, welcoming you to inner space.

3. Give your inner sight a wakeup call. Gently touch the fingertips of your right hand to your forehead, above the eyebrows and between them. Return your hand to your lap.

4. Still keeping your physical eyes closed, turn your inner vision outward towards your reflection in the mirror or towards your partner. Imagine/feel/see the presence of the physical form. Linger over it with your inner vision.

5. Ask to see the aura, and go with whatever experience comes. For best results, be lighthearted about this rather than a perfectionist. Have fun with all the freedom that closed eyes can bring.

6. Consult your inner dictionary as appropriate.

7. Conclude your session of aura reading. Give yourself a couple of minutes for transition time. Then open your eyes.

Toning

Discover how well your subtle hearing works by singing to auras, also known as *toning*. As a side effect, toning perks up the energy within the aura you sing to. Find out how this happens by toning to your own energy field.

1. Prepare the environment. Find a quiet room where you will not be interrupted for ten minutes. Sit in a comfortable chair or lie down.

2. Select one part of your body at a time for toning, for example your rib cage. Gently focus attention on that body part by doing one or more of the following:

   • With your primary sensor hand, rub the aura above the body part. Keep your hand there throughout the toning.

- Close your eyes. Take three vibe-raising breaths. Use inner sight (as described in the previous section) to connect with the body part. Or open your eyes and look at the aura that way.

- Use *mind-body breath*: take a deep breath, consciously aiming the fresh air to the body part. Breathe out as if the air carries away stale energy that was stuck in the body part. Do this for three minutes or longer. You'll feel that body part wake up and start to speak to you intuitively. For several minutes afterwards, your awareness will remain actively connected to the chosen body part, an excellent preparation for toning.

- Crystal power to the rescue! Do you own a single-terminated, clear quartz crystal? Hold it in your primary sensor hand. Point the termination towards your chosen body part. The crystal will act as an energy amplifier.

3. Set the intention to do a *diagnostic toning*, one that will give you information about the energy dynamics of the body.

4. Open your mouth and sing one long note. Sing a vowel sound like "Ah" or "Oh." Don't worry about sounding pretty. The sound might waver in pitch, sound sweet or growly, whatever. Your voice is giving feedback to the energy in that body part right now. Continue to sing more notes until you feel an energy shift, either in the body part or within your awareness.

5. If desired, tone to another body part by repeating Step #4. The tone may sound different or similar. Don't try to control the pitch. Let your Higher Self figure it out. Under these circumstances, you can't sing a wrong note. Continue toning to different body parts for as long as you like. Your toning session could last one minute or one hour.

6. Finish with an auric seal, as explained earlier in this chapter.

Toning

Q. **The singing was fun but what did it have to do with aura reading?**

A. Toning is a deceptively simple technique to develop clairaudience, your subtle sense of hearing. Beyond that, toning can *produce* healing: Feedback to your body energy works like a wakeup call, shifting stuck energy and intensifying healthy patterns.

> **Whenever you deeply acknowledge
> what someone experiences energetically
> without trying to change it,
> you facilitate growth.**

Diagnostic toning to your body's energy gives a direct, spontaneous feedback that is all the more powerful for being nonverbal.

Q. **Is there another form of toning besides diagnostic toning?**

A. Yes, *energy transmission toning*. Its purpose is to send healing energy into the aura to promote and/or stabilize change.

Q. **How do you do it?**

A. Very much like diagnostic toning. Refer to the previous technique for toning but make two changes:

- Instead of using your primary sensor hand, use your alternate sensor hand (otherwise known as your energy blaster).
- As you go through the steps of toning, at Step #3 set an intention to do an energy transmission toning rather than a diagnostic toning.

Q. **Under what circumstances is it helpful to do an energy transmission toning?**

A. Use it after you have moved energy in someone's chakras. (Techniques in this book for doing this include diagnostic toning, auric massage, homeopathy, aromatherapy, flower essences, music, and affirmations.)

Q. How is the energy transmitted?

A. Once you set the intention for energy transmission, your Higher Self automatically selects tones to enliven healthy changes that have taken place in the aura. It's a form of spiritual feedback.

Giving this feedback about the mind-body system through singing these tones is very validating. It could be compared to complimenting someone who has just danced his first waltz. Even the clumsiest version of a waltz deserves recognition, and your encouragement will make future learning easier.

Energy transmission toning reinforces positive auric change as if you said to an awkward new waltzer, "Hey, you're dancing!"

Q. Clairaudience is my strongest subtle sense. How can I make the most of it when doing energy work?

A. Do a diagnostic toning when you start a healing session. Facilitate healing by using clairaudient techniques, such as *guided affirmations* and *healing music.*

Q. Guided affirmations?

A. Follow the basic procedure for toning. At Step #3, ask to hear affirmations that would be conducive to healing for your client. At Step #4, rather than singing, speak the words that come to you. Repeat them aloud as affirmations. Then follow through with the rest of the toning procedure.

Q. **Great! Now how do I do healing music?**

A. Sit as if to read your inner dictionary. Follow the steps of the basic procedure, only this time your "question" will be to sing or play healing music.

After you drop the question and take your vibe-raising breaths, let the music flow. Spontaneously you will create the perfect sound for moving energy. (To learn more about how music moves energy, pay special attention to a later section in Chapter Five on "The Healing Power of Music.")

Q. **Back at regular toning, how can I tell for myself what toning does to my aura?**

A. Take *auric before-and-after pictures.* Before you begin toning, use one of the following methods to read your aura:

- Position your primary sensor hand in front of your body. Choose one or more body parts to investigate, like your throat or solar plexus. Do an aura bounce and aura rub.
- Look at your aura in the mirror.
- Close your eyes. Read your inner dictionary. Your question is, "What is going on with my energy right now?"

After you finish toning, check your aura again, using exactly the same method as before.

Q. **Is this wacky or what? Before each tone came out of my mouth, I heard it inside my head.**

A. That's one form subtle hearing can take. Good for you.

Q. **I love this toning! Now that I have the hang of it, can I do it on people beside myself?**

A. Sure. Just warn them first. Toning makes an excellent follow-up to auric massage.

How to Sing a Smell

Smell and taste make deep and complex impressions on us, even before we delve into subtle aspects of perception. That's because olfactory information is chemical. Odors tell your body directly how they will change your physical system (which will result, of course, in changes to your electromagnetic energy field, your aura).

Here is a basic technique to experience directly how smell and taste transform auras:

Sing that Smell

1. Take an auric before picture, using your primary sensor hand or auravision. Sing the pattern of energy.

2. Smell or taste anything healthy for you—a dill pickle, sandalwood incense, peppermint soap—you name it.

3. Take an auric after picture, using the same technique you used for Step #1. Sing the new pattern of energy.

   What will you learn? Smells can shift an aura. And the fun of this discovery lies in the nuances of your direct experience. As always, God is in the details.

Turn Perfume into a Multimedia Show

Because smell and taste rearrange energy so directly, it's fun to translate their effects on your aura in terms of other senses. Synesthesia helps you do this if you only remember to put in a request.

The following technique is fun because it pulls together so many subtle senses. Another advantage is that this technique depends on smell from the subtle level of synesthesia rather than physical smell. This can be helpful if you don't think your sense of smell is all that great.

1. Assemble several fragrances within reach, three at least, so you can do contrasting readings. Place all the bottles nearby, caps on tight. You'll be reading one fragrance at a time. Also, put art supplies in a convenient place (it's one of the options for Step #4).

2. Place your primary sensor hand within the perfume bottle's auric field and do an aura rub.

   Alternatively, if you're oriented more towards sight than touch, try this technique for *visual touch*.

> **With visual touch you let your sight and synesthesia
> do the feeling. Look at the energy field and
> do an aura bounce and aura rub.
> See? You can touch with your eyes.**

3. Take three vibe-raising breaths.

4. Express your perception of the fragrance.

   • Set an intention to sing the pattern of energy in the perfume's aura. Then just do it. Sing. As described in the previous section on toning, your voice will automatically find the appropriate pitch or pattern of notes to express your subtle perception.

   • Another choice is to express your perception of smell through art. Draw the perfume's dynamic of energy. Crayons, pastels, or markers; one color or many; use whichever medium you wish. Just don't premeditate. Grab the first color that appeals to you and go.

> **Allow yourself to be as spontaneous as a child;
> this will enable you to bypass established
> mental patterns and express a fresher,
> subtler perception.**

5. Explore more deeply. Consult your inner dictionary for more information about the fragrance and what it does to you. Alternatively, use subtle touch to feel directly what the fragrance does to your aura. For example, a violet-based fragrance might open up an area of your aura around the upper body while musk stimulates the aura around the lower part of the body.

6. Now for your reward: After your reading of a perfume is done, open the bottle and smell it. Wow! It's hard to describe in words the surprising perfection of the fragrance you have already "smelled" through other senses.

Especially if you don't much use your physical sense of smell, you owe it to yourself to play with perfume as a multimedia event.

Perfume

Q. **Gustatory giftedness is my clearest form of subtle perception. How can I use it to move energy?**

A. Aromatherapy is a natural for you. After you select the perfect fragrance for yourself or your client, fill the room with it. Take auric before-and-after pictures.

Q. **Hey, I just had a thought. Could I go back to all the earlier techniques (for subtle touch, subtle sight, and so forth) but prepare the environment with a fragrance first?**

A. Excellent idea. Your experiences will be clearer.

Q. **Any other ways to use subtle smell and taste to move energy?**

A. Use subtle smell for "Tantra," discussed in Chapter Five, by smelling each chakra.

Smell while you do the "Heart of the Heart" technique for emotional touch in Chapter Four.

Chapter 4

Explore Chakras

For more advanced aura reading, it helps to know about the structure of the human aura. *Gulp. Suffer through a dry lesson in spiritual anatomy, is that what I'm about to ask you to do?* Never fear. Nothing about this sort of spiritual anatomy need intimidate you. In fact, to put yourself in the right frame of mind, I'd recommend that you travel backwards in time with me, back to your childhood.

Can you remember when you first learned about animals? You discovered that a sheep would bleat, a duck would quack. One animal was soft, fuzzy, and timid; another was quick, brightly colored, able to swim and fly.

Wonder was involved here. You weren't just learning names. Instead you plunged into the experience of a whole cluster of perceptions, maybe even some telepathic connection to the unique consciousness of each kind of animal.

I like to use this analogy in the context of chakras because so many adults use naming as a way to keep out wonder, rather than let it in.

Please don't let the name or concept for a chakra become a substitute for having a rich experience. Each new creature, or chakra, has a kind of life all its own. Naming can be just a beginning.

Mystery comes alive when you connect up with the energy in chakras. Let your sense of wonder be your guide as I take you exploring.

Introducing... The Chakras

Here are some basic definitions to start off your exploration of chakras:

- The energy field around the physical body is the aura as a whole.
- This aura consists of many subtle bodies layered over each other, but to keep matters simple I refer to the whole package as "subtle body."

  Different experts count different numbers of bodies, depending on their specialties as aura readers. You, too, will gravitate towards one or more layers of aura. I'll leave it to your inner dictionary to explain the nuances of different layers. Most important: You only need to perceive one layer of subtle body to do a powerful reading.

- The aura has parts called chakras. Pronounce the first part of the word like "CHOColate" or "SHOCKwave," according to your preference. Both are correct.
- Chakras are places where the subtle body's energy flow is most concentrated. You could make an analogy to organs that govern the systems of the physical body. Just as the physical heart is the center of operations for the body's circulatory system, the heart chakra is the center for the body's higher emotions.

Throughout the world, from time immemorial, people have learned about chakras: Indians—both Eastern and Native American, Africans, Australians, Asians. In Europe, the tradition of bioenergetics also focuses on the subtle body and the chakras.

**Every human body comes complete with
seven main chakras. Each one connects to a different
aspect of being alive, both physically and spiritually.**

But these facts are only the letter of natural law. Your direct experience will reveal the spirit. After all, a duck is more than an aquatic bird. Sheep are more than ruminant mammals of the genus Ovis. Real life critters are alive, lively, individual, always changing, sometimes a little mopey or dopey, other times functioning at a level that is utterly awesome.

That's the story of your chakras, too.

Chakra Specialties

It's fascinating to perceive and interpret what goes on in the different chakras. Each one tells you a specific part of a person's inner truth. For instance:

- Right now Robert is bragging like crazy; inside he feels hopeless and helpless.

- Valerie's trying hard to show how loveable she is, a performance set up for failure because the love-receptor part of her system has shut down.

- Tiffany sits shyly at the edge of the group. Not only does she contribute few words to the conversation, her body language mumbles, "Ignore me." Nevertheless, Tiffany's heart chakra is so strong, it bathes the entire room with light.

Each chakra specializes in a particular part of the truth. These specifics go far beyond beginner's generalizations like "lots of light" or "pink and sparkly." Once you learn the language—and remember, that's *your* way into the language—deep secrets of the chakras will remain secret no longer.

Be a Columbus

Here's your chance to become the Christopher Columbus of the auric realms.

If you have no previous knowledge about chakras, it works to your advantage. Those who already know a little—or a lot—will also benefit from exploring. Put yourself into *beginner's mind*. We're searching a world for subtle spice.

Chakra Probe

1. Ideally, team up with a partner the first time you set out to explore chakras. That way you can take turns being the client. Ask your client to lie down on his back, close his eyes, and use telephone awareness to observe the give-and-take of energy.

   If you can't find a partner, you can explore your own chakras. Please sit those chakras in a chair, rather than laying them down. The explorer's mind will stay clearer that way.

2. Use your primary sensor hand or visual touch to bounce and rub the aura from the head down. Visit the energy over the face. Traverse the trunk. Amble your hand from hips to feet. Meander over each arm. Pay special attention to the *amount* and *quality* of energy. Chakras are where energy is most concentrated. Where do you feel this?

3. If you have a partner, explore both sides of the body, front and back. Do energy centers in the front stick out the other side? Any differ-

ence in quality or amount of energy? Compare the front of one elbow with the back of that elbow.

4. After your exploration is finished, remember to do the auric seal.

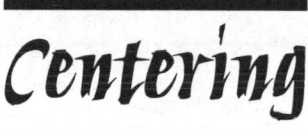

Centering

Since you are advanced enough as an aura reader to explore chakras, consider yourself ready to learn how to center yourself. This is a preparation for energy work and healing. Here are some of the benefits:

- To clear your mind, so you can experience in the here and now.

- To move deeper within, as a reminder to use the subtlest perception of which you are capable.

- To calm down, helping you to do aura reading from a state of balance, even in an emergency.

- To connect to your inner source of wisdom, enabling you to access the most pristine knowledge.

- To gain power from a transpersonal source of healing. If you are about to do energy work, it's imperative to avoid draining yourself. Centering before each client can protect you from this occupational hazard.

Whatever the energy mover's personal problems and limitations, she will do her best when she starts from a state of being centered. And it isn't difficult to do. In practice, the hardest part will be remembering to do it.

A special note to those spiritually-oriented individuals who have resistance to "being in their bodies": centering will ground you there. But your awareness need not stay limited to your physical form. During centering, you may feel a delightful expansion of your awareness that goes far beyond the body. That's a bonus. What matters is that centering fastens your awareness and energy to the physical plane, leading to greater worldly effectiveness.

Even the subtlest perception can be experienced in a centered manner. And the more centered you are, the more effective you will be in using subtle perception to achieve what you desire.

Centering

1. Close your eyes to bring awareness within.

2. Take three vibe-raising breaths.

3. Feel the outline of your physical body. An envelope of skin surrounds you; clothes cover you. Become aware of the dimensions of your body.

4. Feel the contact of your feet with the ground. Intensify that contact by imagining that the soles of your feet are heavy, as though you were stepping in some delightfully thick, sticky mud.

5. Take one or more grounding breaths. Open your eyes.

The Chakras (According to Rose)

Here is the framework I use to read chakras. Prefacing it with my name is intended as a reminder that spiritual truth is relative: one truth per person and nobody owns it all. Even gospel comes in four versions, Matthew, Mark, Luke, and John. So please use the accompanying list of chakras as a starting point for your own research.

I pay close attention to seven main chakras.

Most authorities identify seven of them, but not always in the same locations. Additionally some authorities list a specific color supposed to ideally match each chakra, thus adding another bit to the myth about auras. If God had intended each chakra to have a permanent color, how come we don't have the color coded directly onto our skin?

Until I see some brightly colored polka dots, I'll leave it to you to decide what color each chakra "must" be.

Many systems of energy work involve treating the *sub-chakras* as well as main chakras. Sub-chakras are energy centers in places like the elbows, hands, and knees. Do you need to become involved with this stuff? As a beginning aura reader, and maybe as an advanced one, too, you can get all the knowledge you need from the seven main chakras.

Some energy workers explore additional major chakras, located above the head and other places. Katrina Raphaell, a world-class crystal healer and author, has written about them compellingly. For further study, see her how-to, *The Crystalline Transmission.*

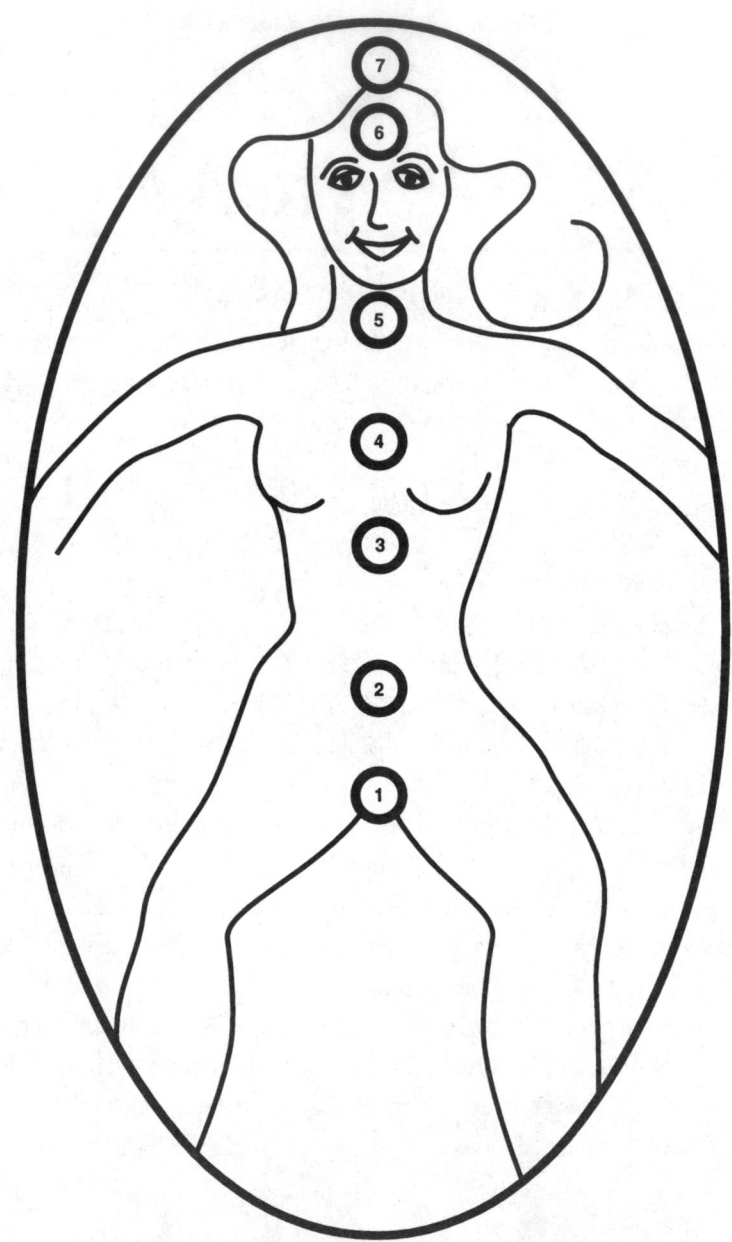

The Seven Main Chakras

Chakra	Location, Seen from the Front
1. Root	The base of the spine
2. Lower Abdominal	Two inches below the navel
3. Solar Plexus	The midriff
4. Heart	Heart level, in the center of the body
5. Throat	The throat, from the collarbone up to the Adam's apple
6. Third Eye	Between the eyebrows and above them
7. Crown	The top of the head

But the primary chakras are of primary importance, and what matters is that you read them to discover your unique perceptions, knowledge, and service.

Therefore, the following section presents some simple but significant tips for reading chakras effectively.

Chakra Reading Tips

1. First Impressions Count

Trust your first impressions about chakras. They will be the truest bits of information available. To some extent, everyone registers this data unconsciously, regardless of training. By the time information trickles over to the conscious mind, though, aura scans typically are reduced to global generalizations, such as "I like her" or "I don't like her."

How much more informative it will be to make the full perception conscious. To some extent aura reading means teasing subconscious impressions out to your conscious mind. What will that take? Curiosity. Trust. A sense of humor wouldn't hurt.

2. Set Aside Judgment

Statements like, "I like her" and "I don't like her" actually have very limited usefulness. Besides, aura reading is not about liking, it's about learning.

**For the deepest and clearest perception,
it helps to approach your subject
with unconditional love.**

---

3. Doubt Your Doubts

Commit to exploring the techniques in this book again and again until any self-doubts are demolished. Doubts are definitely part of the process. And learning to let them go can be a valuable part of your spiritual evolution.

Sure, it is possible to completely avoid any doubt, with all the associated vulnerability and awkwardness. You can go through the following techniques as a skeptic or a speed reader, never letting yourself become deeply involved. By skimming the words you could pick up enough data to pass as a chakra reader. But if you actually use the techniques offered here, doubts will come up, guaranteed. That's the price for a genuine experience.

For some readers, learning to read chakras may be something you wind up doing every day of your life. For other readers, it will be enough to succeed *once* at each technique, expanding the boundaries of what you believe it is possible to know. It's like traveling to a new place for the first time. Whether you go to New York to visit or to live, you will acquire a direct experience that can't be gained any other way.

4. Prepare to Raise Your Vibrations Even Higher

Have your experiences so far amazed you? There is so much more to come.

All the aura reading techniques you have learned so far are powerful and profound. But you will vastly increase their effectiveness when you apply them in the new ways featured in this chapter. Experiencing this can move you further toward celestial consciousness.

5. Use Beginner's Mind

Reading chakras means that you can learn information that is utterly new, different from all you already know about people. Chakras speak a unique language of life energy. This conveys a deeper truth than expression, body language, or other modalities of truth you already use.

Sometimes new chakra readers try to hold onto this old knowledge while they explore what's new. Jumping back and forth between these two ways of knowing results in confusion more than clarity.

You'll do better to let go of old knowledge and explore the level of chakras with beginner's mind. Start fresh to put yourself into the here and now.

The appropriate time to shift gears from one kind of knowledge to another is *after*, not *during*, a session of chakra reading.

6. Responsibility Comes With This Privilege

Knowledge is power. Chakra knowledge intensifies your power to learn some of life's closely held secrets. But privilege and responsibility must go together. That is why the more deeply you delve into aura reading the greater becomes your moral responsibility to do no harm.

Don't fall into the trap of using aura reading for personal gain rather than service. *Negative consequences for others* can include causing spiritual confusion for which they, and ultimately you, will pay a price. *Negative consequences for yourself* can include having your spiritual development screech to a halt.

For instance, Ellen used her clairvoyance to show off. After she started seeing auric colors, Ellen got into the habit of bragging about it to her friends. She wanted the status of being considered "spiritually gifted." Ellen never considered that by bragging she might discourage her friends from developing their own subtle senses. And it never occurred to Ellen that this "proof" of her spiritual superiority could hold back her own progress.

Years after Ellen began doing this, we had a heart-to-heart talk. She complained that although she continued to see colors, her ability to interpret them had not developed one iota. Even worse, she bemoaned the fact that, despite hours of meditation each day, she had been spiritually stuck for at least five years.

7. Be Clear About Your Motivation

Unless you pause to consciously consider your motivation, you may forget about service to others. Upgrade your aura reading by choosing to serve others with respect and genuine helpfulness.

One definition of helpfulness is to give what the other person needs rather than what you have in excess.

How can you best help your friend John when you become a chakra reader? No matter how clear your intuition, don't try to play God by anticipating his needs. Ask John to tell you directly if he wants a reading.

Even the right words, offered at the wrong time, can backfire. It's like a wonderful old proverb: *Speak only the sweet truth.* Part of the truth can be hurtful rather than sweet. How much good will it do to tell it? Unless you're dealing with matters of life or death, don't waste your words.

Motivation really matters when you are helping others. Desire to provide loving help. Your inspiration will flow deeper. Lesser desires, like making people admire you, can taint wisdom. If you have ever noticed "ego flavor" in help from others, you'll know the mixed results on the receiving end.

8. Purity of Heart

Another problem with misuse of aura reading involves clarity. Take the case of Mike, who enjoyed part-time income as a professional psychic. To interest prospective clients, Mike would drop little hints in the form of *vanity feedings,* like "Did you know that your aura is unusually large?"

Clients came Mike's way, of course, but his readings became increasingly inaccurate. Mike distorted his channels for subtle knowing by doing what, deep down, he knew to be wrong.

What you will discover is that your clarity as an aura reader develops in direct proportion to your purity of heart. Resolve to use your readings only for good.

How else can you keep your heart pure?

- Tell people the truth when you talk to them.
- Be willing to *hear* the truth, too. Listen for the whole truth. Denial never helped anyone to advance spiritually.
- Look for beauty rather than dwelling on faults.
- Whenever possible, associate with others who have pure hearts.
- Avoid exposing yourself to hatred and sensationalism.
- Judge others, if you must judge them at all, by the same lenient standard you accord your own motives.
- Honor your commitments. Don't take on more than you can handle.
- Set ethical standards for yourself as an aura reader. Set them now.

Ethics

Nobody has the right to dictate what your ethics should be, but it will be in your best interests to set a high standard.

Don't assume that your ability to delve into chakras constitutes an open invitation. This stuff couldn't be more personal.

As you become increasingly familiar with auras, a certain amount of information will present itself wherever you go. But choice is always there. When the book opens to you, will you choose to read it or move on?

Situational ethics apply. To illustrate, I'll tell you when this chakra reader feels it is right to actively do detective work:

- For security purposes when among strangers I do a quick scan for outrageously dysfunctional auras and chakras. My inner alarm will register major anger, hatred, craziness, etc. When the siren goes off, I cross the street or leave the room.

- For truth in relationships, chakra reading is unsurpassed. It's fair to keep tabs on those you love.

  Major withholds show in the chakras, as you'll read later in detail. Debra was knocked for a loop when she discovered her husband had been unfaithful to her for six months. If she had known how to check in with his chakras on a regular basis, Debra would have seen something was wrong. Behavior, words, and body language can be manipulated. Chakras can't (except in the case of a truly world class actor).

- To be the best friend possible, use chakra knowledge for deep listening to what is really going on. "How are you?" can be asked conversationally or for in-depth sharing. Depending on the level of answer you seek, you may choose to read chakras.

What if someone you love is going through a difficult time but keeps up a stoic front? For instance, Keisha's behavior gave no clue to the outside world of how bad she felt. But her chakras revealed to me that she was deeply depressed. I shared with her what I had noticed, asking if it was true and offering to help. The validation alone meant a great deal to her.

- Development of celestial consciousness is a legitimate motive for reading anyone's chakras, so long as the reading is kept private. After all, the difference between spiritual seeking and gossip can hang on a word—whether it is spoken or kept silent.

Be sure to read chakras of those who are especially gifted, be they musicians, politicians, teachers, an undercover saint in the form of your local reference librarian ... any potential source of inspiration.

- For entertainment, read auras of professional entertainers. Actors, athletes, TV journalists, and such have chosen to put their chakras on display. I believe it is fair game to observe them, even to talk about them. By contrast, what right do I have to gossip about the chakras belonging to the guy in front of me on line at the supermarket? I'd better have pretty good reason to discuss him. Idle curiosity would be better confined to the contents of the man's shopping cart.

Some chakras inspire. Some show mistakes to avoid. Especially important, chakras often help an aura reader to understand behavior that otherwise would seem inexplicable. Your sense of humor is going to get better and better. That's a serious promise!

Deep Chakra Reading

Now is your chance to check out the chakras more clearly than ever before. Test out the seven chakra positions I have presented, starting with number one, the root. Also retest any energy centers you found on your own that do not correspond to my list. A detailed understanding about each chakra will unfold in the rest of this chapter and is summarized later. Nevertheless, theoretical knowledge about the chakras is not necessary for you to read them. For best results approach them with beginner's mind.

Use any of the sensing methods you've learned, alone or in combination. Consult with your inner dictionary. Examine chakras on yourself or a partner. One interesting question to ask is whether the chakra seems strong or weak.

A Strong Chakra

A strong chakra feels like it has a lot of energy. If you are doing an aura bounce you may have to reach quite a distance from the body before you make contact with the outside of the energy field.

When you rub the energy, you may receive a vibrant texture or temperature. You'll feel something lively, pulsating, bouncy—something your inner dictionary registers as positive.

To see a chakra, look at the aura over the body part where the chakra is located. A strong chakra shows a lot of light. If you see a color, the color will be clear or bright. If you see textures, notice how the texture is lively, sparkly, etc.

Chakras are made of moving energy. Hands or eyes may give you a sense of this movement. Or use a tea bag as tool. With thumb and forefinger, hold a dry tea bag by the paper tag. Position it about four inches from the body at the place where the chakra is located.

At first the tea bag will dangle, motionless, from the string. Soon it will begin to move in a pattern that corresponds to the flow of chakra energy. Probably it will move in a clockwise direction (or counterclockwise if you're in the southern hemisphere). Pretty impressive!

A strong chakra is a pleasure to tone. Your voice sounds attractive, connected, strong.

Touching, seeing, and toning are not the only methods you will find helpful for reading chakras.

> **Remember that you can combine your subtle senses;**
> **it's valid because they are connected by synesthesia.**
> **So, while looking, you can ask:**
> **"What does this chakra tell me?"**
> **"What emotions are in this chakra now?" and so forth.**

Depending on your spiritual gifts, you could receive an intense emotion, feel a physical sensation right in your own body, smell a fragrance, taste a flavor. Information can also come to you directly, either by hearing words from inside or a sense of direct knowing. One way or another, healthy chakras send out a message that is positive.

A (Temporarily) Weak Chakra

Any chakra belonging to a live body can be repaired, but sometimes you'll find them in pretty bad shape. In that case, an aura bounce may reveal little energy. An aura rub may show something funny going on with the texture, like brittleness or coldness.

Visually, you may find little light. Colors may be dull, with dark spots or blobs, tears or tears. And just as these two t-words gave you pause, chakra problems grab your attention. You'll stumble over a listless lack of pep or come to a screeching halt, as if at a stop sign that reads TROUBLE. Sixth sense knowledge may give you specifics about what the trouble is. Your inner dictionary certainly can, so don't forget to use it when confronted with a chakra in distress.

You also might choose to ask your dictionary how you can be of service.

But how much of this information is appropriate to tell, especially when the news is bad? Tact alert! It's better not to scare people. My solution is to give limited, low-key summaries about problems I pick up in the chakras. My goal is to supply just enough detail and intensity to validate what a client already feels. However, I avoid sharing bad news unless I am also prepared to *help*.

Chapter Five contains many techniques for healing the chakras. But before you go on to explore them, use the rest of this chapter to deepen your knowledge of the individual chakras.

Being Human

Just because you're a human being doesn't mean you like being human. The first chakra reveals, at any given moment, the degree of safety you feel about living on this planet in human form. Actually, the root chakra shows many facets of a person's relationship to physicality.

To find the first chakra from the front, follow the legs up to the crotch. As with all chakras, the back view is in the corresponding place on the other side. So for the posterior view of the first chakra, you would check out the tip of the tailbone.

What will you turn up when you explore your root chakra? If it's healthy, you'll find:

- A baseline feeling of security, psychological wellbeing
- Content-ability (as opposed to the feeling of never receiving enough attention, love, money, etc.)
- Trust that your significant others will respond to your needs
- A welcoming attitude towards new people in your life
- Acceptance of your physical body, a healthy self-image
- Comfort with your sexual orientation, whatever it may be
- Groundedness, connection with all of physical life

Thus, the first chakra can serve as the foundation for a mature, well adjusted personality. By contrast, clients with major root chakra problems may be chronically suspicious, tense, or spaced out. Addictions, eating disorders, and sexual shutdown can also relate to malfunction at the level of the first chakra. Problems here have shown up in my counseling clients whose history includes an alcoholic parent, child abuse, incest, or rape.

That's the bad news. The good news is that every step of progress makes the chakra stronger, helping a person to become more secure, deep down.

First Chakra Fun

Check out the first chakra of every child you can.

1. Use your primary sensor hand or auravision to read the root chakra.
2. Consult your inner dictionary for interpretation.
3. Give a brief aura massage. Babies love it.
4. Close with an auric seal.

Happy infants, toddlers, and preschoolers show the most delectable flavors of trust. Young auras are usually an inspiration all around, but the root chakra of a well-adjusted child is a special delight.

Coming on to You?

Someone is looking you over. Nobody can be caught staring. Yet somehow you know you're being assessed as a desireable cut of meat.

How do you know?

The Beach Boys called it "Good Vibrations." The words to their golden oldie make a lot more sense when you realize they're really about vibes in the second chakra, not the totality of a person. This part of the human energy system is set up to receive, transmit, and acknowledge sexual messages.

You'll find the lower abdominal chakra about two inches below the navel. And isn't it convenient that you, the aura reader, can delve into this highly personal chakra with nothing more obvious than a quick but probing glance.

The second chakra offers information about more than sex, too. It clues you in to how lively someone's Inner Child may be, the playfulness and creativity. Intuitive ability also shows up in a strong second chakra. Think about it. All these aspects of life are connected.

Primal emotions, too, reveal themselves at the second chakra. Should you need a reminder of their passionate vividness, babysit any two year old. When these emotions flow freely, life is intense. At least denial isn't a problem.

What happens, though, when the second chakra doesn't function so well? Sex becomes ho-hum or empty ... or obsessively important. Creativity drops away from the rest of living. A stifled Inner Child lives the form of relationships without the content, motions without meaning.

Sexual Detective Work

What will he or she be like in bed? If you'd like a preview—and assuming you can't find out all you need to know by observing how your intended drives a car—the second chakra is your best source of information. Detective work is simple. The only difficulty is doing it discretely.

1. Choose your subject. (Remember your ethics, please. Make sure you have good reason to snoop.)

2. Mentally, ask for information about what your subject is like sexually.

3. Take a quick look at the second chakra. Use subtle sight with your eyes open or closed.

4. Immediately avert your eyes. This gives you privacy to sort out what you have seen.

> **When you don't touch the aura at close range,
> you can explore at length without the need
> to follow up with an auric seal.**

In most circumstances, using your primary sensor hand is out of the question (unless you want to make your curiosity rather obvious). But even if, like me, you're more a feeler than a seer, there is a technique for using your eyes to touch auras. It's great in cases like this where discretion would be appropriate ... or if for any reason you can't get close enough to physically touch an aura.

Touchy Sight

This technique uses the power of synesthesia to open up deeper sight.

1. Direct your eyes to the spot where you would apply your primary sensor hand if you could.

2. Playfully imagine that you are physically touching.

   - One way to do this is to visualize a light body within your physical body: move it away from the rest of you, walk it over to your subject, and touch the aura with your primary sensor hand.

   - Another technique is to stay fully in your body but mentally agree that where you look will be tantamount to touching.

For practice, visit an art museum. Don't just look at the paintings. Touch them with your eyes until you feel that you can walk around in them.

Once you master touchy sight, it will provide the same kind of information that comes through the primary sensor hand: amount of energy, texture, feeling, and so forth.

Believe me, when someone comes on to you energetically, you'll find plenty to watch. If that person's desire is strong enough to show in verbal or nonverbal ways, the second chakra will come on double strong. It's quite a spectacle.

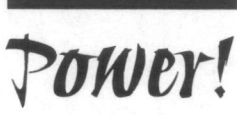

Power!

The solar plexus chakra is your power center. When it is healthy, you know what you want and feel confident about going for it. If provoked to fight, you expect to win.

Besides that, a healthy third chakra helps you hold your ground. Blaming isn't necessary. You can accept full responsibility for your life.

Unique among all the chakras, number three actually changes location when chronically malfunctioning. If you don't make contact with chakra energy in the center of the body between the waistline and rib cage, move your primary sensor hand to the person's left, just above the waistline, all the way over to the side of the body.

Some energy workers have encountered the third chakra in this location so often, they refer to it as The Spleen Chakra.

Spleen. Associate that word with ill temper? Got that right. Prolonged powerlessness doesn't go with a sunny disposition.

Power center problems translate into phrases like "I can't," "Why bother?" "I don't know what I want," and "Poor me."

A mild case? Butterflies in the stomach come and go. Chronic problems? Worry becomes a habit. Digestive ailments may enter the picture.

Even if you're a staunch believer in affirmations, don't expect affirmations alone to fix third chakra problems—except for those aforementioned butterflies. The person needs therapy, energy work, something. The type of professional help must match the patient's belief system, of course, for any lasting healing to take place.

A Word to the Wise: Attention

Americans today are obsessed with deception and it's easy to understand why. In our current phase we're collectively learning more about the third chakra than any other. Violence and victimization, in all its shades of melodrama, are presented as a form of light entertainment. Not surprisingly, we feel an acute need to protect ourselves from liars and cheats ... to such an extent that self-protection can become a full-time job, if you let it.

Perspective, though, comes from remembering an important law of nature. Attention changes life. In physics this law operates as Heisenberg's Uncertainty Principle. Spiritually, it's a law of attraction.

Whatever you pay attention to grows stronger in your life.

Beyond taking reasonable precautions, or satisfying your curiosity, emphasis on deception can poison a life. Please don't use aura reading to make yourself a magnet for the world's ills.

All this notwithstanding, I must tell you that aura reading is a superb method to gauge a truthful character.

One way to use it is for routine checkups of your significant other and close family members, as mentioned earlier; other techniques are supplied in this chapter. Right now I'll share with you one of my favorite techniques for self-protection.

Warning Bells

1. Before going into a situation where someone's deception may place you at risk, set an intention that an intuitive warning bell will go off as appropriate. Ask in terms of your strongest spiritual gift. For instance:

- Tom has asked to hear a ring in the voice of anyone trying to trick him.

- Donna has asked to be shown auric symbols. When she sees auras, wiggles indicate slippery tactics, dark spots show *psychic coercion* (a control drama where one person tries to force another person's will).

- Steve has asked for truth knowledge to interrupt the usual flow of consciousness the way TV shows say, "We interrupt this broadcast for a fast-breaking news bulletin."

2. Once your attention has been alerted to possible deception, drop whatever else you're doing and find out what's going on. Read the person's power center. This is your single most vital chakra for information about deception.

3. Use your favorite technique to tune into the power center. Especially effective modalities for this are auravision, touchy sight, physical empathy, and truth knowledge. Ask, "What is going on here in terms of truthfulness?" The results may amaze you.

Liars and Cheats on Parade

Without the kind of deep knowledge available from chakras, discerning deception is hard work. For example, it takes a lot of effort to keep your eyes trained on the face for telltale nonverbal clues, like giveaway eye movement. (Did you know that just before a right-handed person tells a whopper, eyes shift to the left, and vice versa for a left-handed person? Interesting concept, but try to catch the flicker. It flies by pretty fast.)

Truth Technique #1

Instead of constant surveillance for nonverbal clues, try this simple method.

1. Choose a person to examine.

2. Use auravision or touchy sight to look at the solar plexus chakra.

3. Ask inwardly to be shown if that person is centered or, more precisely, *how* that person is centered. Insights will come to you. For clarification, consult your inner dictionary.

Beyond Body Language

By comparison with Truth Technique #1, information from nonverbal communication is not only harder to find, it's less reliable.

For example, an expert at nonverbal communication may have taught you to listen for the pitch of a speaker's voice. Uncentered speech comes out higher in pitch than a person's regular speaking voice. But why?

- Alex may simply be embarrassed by the topic of the conversation.
- Carly may speak with a high-pitched voice because she was taught long ago it is "the feminine way" to ask for things.
- Christopher's voice may trail upwards in pitch in feeble protest of his victimhood. Wimpy? Yes. Dishonest? No.

Auras can uncover secrets that tell you more than a global generalization like "uncentered." Alex and Carly's chakras, for instance, show nothing important going on, truthfulness-wise. Poor Christopher's power center reveals a donut-like hole. But none of these auras turns up a real problem, like the spikes of aggressiveness or the slime of deception.

To complete a thorough hunt for lies, you'll want to supplement power center readings with watching the throat chakra, as discussed later. But the search for integrity should still start with the power center. The worst lies are those that are lived, not just spoken.

Emotional Truth

Heart chakras specialize in deep emotional truth. They show a person's pattern of giving love and—just as revealing—the extent to which a person allows love to be received.

You'll find the fourth chakra heart-level in the center of the body— and on a man's body, right between the nipples. Depending on how a woman is built, the nipples may be located nearer the solar plexus chakra, so a better guide is to find the chakra between the shoulder blades.

Emotion, that's what this chakra reveals. But it's not the raw, primal feelings of the second chakra. Rather, the fourth chakra specializes in "higher" emotions like love, spiritual yearning, and compassion. One way to appreciate the difference relates to the temperature of tears.

Have you ever noticed, some tears are hot? They release second chakra feelings like anger. Cold tears, by contrast, signify the melting of the heart, fourth chakra emotional purification. Cold tears can well up over the plight of other people. Hot tears are always about ME, ME, ME.

Healthy heart chakras reveal openheartedness, the capacity to love, friendliness given freely, a sense of worthiness about accepting love from others, and last but not least, *genuine* self-love.

What kind of self-love would not be genuine? Bogus forms of self-love do exist. Aurically they show up outside the heart chakra.

- Extra energy in the second chakra can denote sexual self-indulgence, rather than balanced self-love.

- Pushy energy at the solar plexus means trying too hard, not self-confidence or self-love.

- A frenzy of energy at the throat can reveal egotism, which bears only the most superficial resemblance to self-love.

When you find a truly happy heart chakra, read it to *your* heart's content. More often, though, this chakra will show sadness, bitterness, and other painful emotions. Whatever walls your subject has built to hide his vulnerability crumble when you read his heart.

Even when these walls of defensiveness are thick, clients can be grateful when an aura reader pays a call, especially if the reader offers sincere encouragement. Once I was invited to comment on the aura of a 14-year-old girl. Jessica was one of many guests at a party where I had been hired to give brief readings. Mostly I was breezing through solar plexus and throat chakras. (Teenagers usually have a delightful spunkiness there. They love to hear me describe their particular flavors of rebelliousness.)

Jessica came last. In tone and body language, she blended so well with the jolly group that I was totally unprepared for what her aura revealed. Limp and listless energy seeped out of most chakras. As for the poor kid's heart chakra, it had more energy than all the chakras below it combined. And what a horrible quality that was—disappointment, a nightmarish sense of betrayal. The self-love part of her heart chakra was in especially deep trouble.

Gently I took Jessica aside to acknowledge her experience. Her eyes overflowed with healing tears.

Depths of the Heart

Heart chakra information will amaze any sensitive aura reader. Wrap perception around the fourth chakra with clairvoyance, emotional touch, or touchy sight. To say you will get a reading is to put it mildly. For empaths it can feel as though being jet propelled into the client's emotional body. And if you're not an empath yet, keep reading heart chakras and you may well become one.

**Don't reserve the treat of heart chakra reading
for people you already love.
Listen to the hearts of people you dislike.
Petty conflicts will melt like Popsicles® in July.**

Even the most obnoxious fool has yearnings that you have shared at one time or another. And often the greatest vulnerability is found in those whose annoying behavior keeps others at a distance. The heart chakra will help you discover a deeper truth.

That truth is sometimes simple. But other times the truth of the heart can build up into very complex patterns. Be prepared to find unexpected mixtures. One heart, at one time, could combine recklessness, shyness, jealousy, self-hatred, and Valentine's Day-sweet romance. Complexity like this makes the heart chakra fascinating.

Beyond all ways of reading heart chakras, I have developed one favorite technique, The Heart of the Heart. (Thanks are due to my co-discoverer, Jeffrey Chappell, a composer, pianist, clairaudient, and emotional empath.) Instructions may seem deceptively simple:

The Heart of the Heart

1. Choose a client. Ask permission in advance for what you want to do, for this technique is hardly inconspicuous.

2. Center yourself.

3. Take three vibe-raising breaths.

4. Put your ear to your client's chest and listen to the heartbeat. That's right, physically listen to the heart.

5. As you hear the heartbeat, set the intention to listen as deeply as possible.

6. Let go, not directing your consciousness one way or another. Let it float. But don't be surprised if your client's heartbeat projects you straight into his deep vibrational frequencies.

7. Take your ear off your friend's chest. Return your consciousness to your personal identity, the familiar sense of being you. For extra grounding, feel where your feet make contact with the floor.

The Heart of the Heart technique enables you to taste the energetic flavor of another person's unique way of being and loving. Practice, relaxation, and willingness can bring on an experience of *spiritual unity*.

Spiritual unity means you experience directly the nature of another person's vibrations, discovering from the inside out how it feels to live—whether on a mental plane—as a pristine fairylike innocence—rigidly grounded, and so forth. You can feel, as though within your own skin, another person's emotional tightness, buried pain, joyfulness ... the works.

The more hearts you listen to, the more you will witness the exquisite beauty of love in all its variations. What a privilege!

Communication Central

Some have a way with words, others express more nonverbally, but all of us manage to communicate somehow. The number of nuances easily exceeds the 1,600 different colors that experts say a human being can see. Even a newborn baby, able to do little to communicate but cry, conveys a wide range of requests and emotions.

When an infant can express such a variety of information—even before knowing that she has a voice for hollering or tiny fists with which to beat the air—imagine how the scope of communication increases over time.

Imagine, but don't bet any money!

Until I started reading **the chakra located at the center and base of the throat**, I had no idea how rare it was to find one in really good shape.

Sure folks are skilled at speaking, and have developed many ways to say what they mean. But often the words are not congruent with deeper reality. Detached from inner truth, the most impassioned shows of speech amount to sound and fury, signifying nothing.

That's the bad news. The good news is that the throat chakra, like all the others, can improve to a state of wonderful balance. In fact, this chapter includes an amazingly simple technique that can reduce your throat chakra clutter by as much as 50% within 24 hours.

But first, how will you recognize a great throat chakra when you (eventually) find one? As with any part of the aura, the clues are brightness, clarity, color, size, carats. Oops, I snuck that part in from an ad for a diamond sale. Just so you don't feel as though you're reading one more of life's endless lists, let's stop right here. It's your turn to talk: how would a great throat chakra sound/feel/look/smell?

Spontaneity, deliberateness, wit, humor, intelligence, music, tunefulness, truthfulness, POWER. Qualities like these are good to keep in mind, because more often than not you'll find a throat chakra with the visual equivalent of a stutter.

Why? Every polite person has been trained to not say certain things. We had to be. Remember how kids talk? "Mr. Hansen, why are you fat?" "Gee, Mrs. Jones, you look so old. How come you're not dead yet?"

For the sake of social survival, every talker becomes a speech squelcher (except for brats, rewarded for their candor, or nastiness, with contempt). Most of us become good little boys or girls with stuffed up throats.

Besides that, throat chakras store our unexpressed pain at not being understood or successful. When we don't dare to express our vulnerability, it doesn't go away; it stays stuck and shadows the throat energy. Sometimes throats even are blocked out of modesty. Did you ever hide a talent so you wouldn't seem like a showoff?

For all these reasons and more, throat chakra readings are guaranteed to stretch your compassion. An unrelated benefit of snooping on throats is convenience. Nobody ever got slapped in the face for watching a throat, especially since your subject will probably think you are riveted on the loveliness of his face. A final bonus is that occasionally you'll be lucky enough to meet a rare and radiant healthy throat chakra, blooming like a hothouse orchid.

Glorious flowers and paintings and music and chakras share one practical thing in common. When you actively soak up whatever makes them glorious, it works like a chiropractic adjustment on your own aura. For a while you become aligned. You could call it spiritual darshan, "healthy contagiousness," or simply "learning by example."

Whatever you call it, do it. Let your subtle perception linger over healthy throat chakras.

Clearing Your Throat

Here's my (formerly) secret formula to clear up a clogged throat chakra:

Speak your truth.

Simple? Yes. But for this to work, you must do it unfailingly on a regular basis, preferably starting as soon as you understand the concept. (That means NOW.)

What's so important about speaking the truth? Unless you're under oath, most people today don't expect you to speak the truth, the whole truth, and nothing but the truth. Sad! But for a healthy throat chakra, you've got to speak at least some of the truth every time.

Speaking the truth means avoiding lies, whether by omission or commission. The Watergate coverup-type whoppers, being highly demanding to keep up, are relatively easy to avoid. Omission lies are trickier.

For instance, you don't have to tell Mr. Hansen what you think of his girth. Nobody asked. But what if, while your family is at his backyard barbecue, he says, "Help yourself to several more servings of roast pork. We know that all the propaganda about health food is a lot of hooey. Cholesterol is good for you, right!"

If you agree, you need say nothing. Your throat chakra can frolic as you keep downing platefuls of pig. But if you disagree, it will rankle that your agreement has been implied. Unless you say something, polite silence will lard up your throat chakra for the next few hours or longer.

So come to your throat's rescue. You need not climb on a soapbox and give the definitive anti-barbecue speech. A tactful "I don't think so," will do, or a quiet "Speak for yourself, Howie Hansen." The point is, speak enough of your truth so it doesn't stay bottled up inside you like fermenting cider.

Incidentally, gossip doesn't work. To keep your throat clear you must speak directly to the person. Use a confrontation, a phone call, a letter. You can even tear the letter up after writing it, but first read your words out loud with expression, as though face-to-face with the one you need to talk to. Your throat chakra will thank you.

Truth Technique #2

Here's a final throat chakra technique expressly for those who are still fascinated by the idea of using aura reading for lie detector tests.

**Lies show in the throat chakra as patterns.
Don't expect every single prevarication
to show up as an auric blob, instantly visible,
like the length of Pinocchio's nose.**

---

1. To find chronic fibbing, look your suspect right in the neck. Use auravision, touchy sight, truth knowledge, or (if you have the luxury) clairsentience with your primary sensor hand.

2. Should you perceive the throat chakra imbalance of "not speaking truth," beware that it can take different forms. So pursue your perception. Look carefully through the use of whichever subtle sense comes most easily. Then consult your inner dictionary. You will come to distinguish throat problems like discouragement, shyness, pain at not being heard. Then there's the ugly sight of chronic lying—more accurately, chronic patterns of hiding the truth.

3. Put your findings in context. After you check the throat, read the solar plexus chakra. Interpret them together.

Returning to the example of Mr. Hansen as he loudly extols the virtues of pork, his speechifying may drive everyone nuts, regardless of dietary preference. When someone's chattering drives *you* nuts, that's a perfect reason to peek at the throat chakra.

Hansen's is probably revved up into overdrive. So look at the starting motor, the solar plexus. With Howie Hansen, the third chakra is a mess. Now you know why his speech is loud in sound, inaudible on impact. The poor guy's words fade into thin air because, aurically, that's what they're made of.

Unfortunate? Yes. Malevolent? No.

By contrast, the relatively few people I've seen whom I would call wicked have color-coordinated yuck lodged in throat and solar plexus, and an even worse version at the third eye (the chakra we'll turn to next).

Special advice for the guilt ridden: Not to worry—it's unlikely that you will ever find three-fold evil in your chakras. The people who have it are more likely to ridicule auras than read them.

How Enlightenment Shows

Many of us know where the "third eye" is located, between the eyebrows and slightly above them, but we don't know what it shows.

Myth has it that the third eye is somehow closed until it a person becomes spiritually enlightened. Then the third eye pops open, like a traffic light turned suddenly and irrevocably green.

But actually spiritual opening is a matter of degree. And this chakra does not simply represent a test of who has completed training and, thus, won't have to repeat another session at Earthling Karmic Junior High. Instead this chakra reveals a person's receptivity to see the spiritual truth. Like charity, receptivity to truth begins at home. Is a man willing to see his current self, the quality of his everyday consciousness?

When healthy, a third eye contains vibrant energy, sometimes lots of it. True, the energy and light of this chakra can have a soul-stirring quality. Cosmic consciousness, celestial consciousness—witnessing auras with these attainments is the highest privilege. Nevertheless, everyone's sixth chakra has something to teach you about spiritual growth-in-progress.

These evolving third eyes show spiritual strain in numerous ways. Fear shows on the forehead of many a righteous believer. When someone insists she knows all about truth and God, observe her third eye for yourself. The news may not be as good as she thinks.

Probably the most common problem involves feeling "holier than thou." Take Nathan, for instance. When his wife hauled him off to a marriage counselor, he saw no point in discussing specifics, like his financial transgressions or extramarital affairs. Instead, he lectured his wife on her "obvious" spiritual shortcomings.

That's third eye junk in action. And it's tempting to laugh at it. But I've pulled some Nathan's in my life and, if you're a spiritual seeker type, chances are that you have too. Spiritually motivated people are most vulnerable to over-interpreting reality, mind control through cults, denial, religious fanaticism. Others can see so clearly what it is. But, in the words of an ancient proverb, *the eyes can't see the eyes.*

An aura reader can, at least, read the spiritual eye.

A Spiritual Checkup

1. Surprisingly, the best way to check on overall spiritual functioning is not to focus on the third eye but to compare and contrast *all* the chakras up to and including it. Start with the root and work your way up. Use clairsentience with your primary sensor hand, truth knowledge, auravision, or touchy sight.

2. Ask questions while you use subtle perception:

   • From one chakra to the next, does the energy match up?

   • Does one chakra bulge out with extra vim, another show no vigor at all?

   • Worst of all, do you find a dull spot where a vibrating chakra ought to be?

3. Consult your inner dictionary. Major imbalance need not be interpreted as a sign of spiritual failure but rather as a warning. That person's spiritual direction may not be as perfect as she thinks. Growth is immanent. The question becomes, will growth come through choice or through drama?

> **When a person is spiritually stuck, change will come.**
> **But how? Will it be through spiritual reassessment,**
> **undertaken voluntarily?**
> **Or will spirit find no alternative but to manifest crises**
> **of finances, health, or other so-called "accidents"?**
> **One way or another growth must come.**

Why not examine your own spiritual life with a chakra checkup? Examining others can help you too, bringing you an extra measure of humility and compassion. Everyone's energy centers have been bumped and bruised. It's a rare being who strides the earth with all chakras drenched in bliss.

Many spiritually-oriented people have magnificent higher chakras: huge power from the heart, dazzling third eyes and crowns, maybe even pretty good throats. But the humble root chakra wilts like an unwatered plant, second chakra energy has evidently gone somewhere on vacation. Sometimes everything bounces with vitality but the power center.

That's life on The Learning Planet! You, the aura reader, are privileged to watch.

And sometimes gratitude for that privilege will hit home in a dramatic way. I remember once being asked to read the aura of an eight-year old boy who was deaf. The way his mother asked for the reading, I knew she badly needed upliftment; I figured it would be easy to find something kind to say.

Some people with disabilities have extraordinary chakras. Even though the energy field is low around the disabled part, like ears or eyes, energy in other areas more than makes up for it. I've heard it said that souls line up for the chance to live in a disabled body because the potential for learning is so great. Auras demonstrate the high consciousness of many who wear these bodies.

Unfortunately, the boy whose aura I was asked to read seemed like a real loser. Physically, Taylor looked tired, skinny, and frail. His face was unattractive, his expression blank, and no glow animated his eyes. The boy had the body language of someone who didn't connect well with others and empathically he was out of reach.

I've read auras of people who were empathically inaccessible for a variety of reasons: being reluctant to have a reading, suspicious, frightened, cold, selfish, deeply depressed, all sorts of reasons. But with this boy it was different. It felt to me that he barely knew how to connect to people, which was tremendously sad.

Without doubt, it was the hardest reading I had ever been asked to do.

Taylor could read my lips, I was told, if only I would speak slowly. Somehow or other I had to come up with a reading. The pressure was on.

Gamely I scanned his chakras, looking for the best news I could tell him and his mother. Starting from his power center up, the tidings were mediocre at best, when whammo! I came to his third eye. It stretched like a Great Wall of China, blasting out an ineffable love.

I realized that this boy was here to be a light of spiritual truth, little more. The other chakras functioned only enough to keep him alive. He was a kind of saint, remarkable not for what he did but for who he was.

How could I express this? We were at a company picnic, not church. I was decked out in a silly gypsy costume to please my client, who had hired me to provide light entertainment. For the sake of my own throat chakra, I would have to express at least some of my truth, but how? I took a deep breath, then asked my inner dictionary for words. There weren't a lot of them but at last they came.

"His spiritual energy is exceptionally strong," I told Taylor's mother. Then I turned to him. "When you look at people, you see what is inside on the outside, don't you?" A brilliant light of understanding flashed in his eyes. For the first time, he smiled.

This world is full of spiritual teachers in disguise. Some of those disguises are pretty thick, but still the auras shine through.

Your Crowning Glory

No it's not your hair, despite what they suggest in the glossy magazine ads. Considering the sequence of your seven glorious energy centers, the one on top should qualify for the title of Crowning Glory. Still it tells less than you might expect, considering what it does.

Where there's life, there's an aura. As long as you live, light pours into that aura. It is spiritual and psychic source energy and it pours in right through the top of your head.

You can find the crown chakra by looking about three inches above the head or by placing your primary sensor hand there for an aura rub.

Don't try an aura bounce because the levels of crown chakra energy go on and on for a huge distance, each progressively more subtle and linked with more universal forms of identity. Perceiving the crown several feet away, one's perception therefore becomes vague. Right above the head, the texture is more readable.

Crown energy, nevertheless, feels pretty much the same for everyone: no more individual than breathing. Like breathing, it's miraculous when you think about it but not terribly fascinating otherwise, which is most of the time.

Not only is the crown chakra relatively dull to read, it won't deliver much insight into a subject's spirituality. Instead, look/feel at the third eye, then at all the chakras below it, as described in the section on "Spiritual Checkup."

The practical point is this: for personal spirituality, read the third eye; the crown shows a more cosmic side of it. Nevertheless, when you're an advanced aura reader, energy from the head on up can take on a new significance.

Group Body

Have you ever heard of the concept called "group body"? It opens up a way for your consciousness to connect with that of other people whenever you are in a group. For a simple example, let's say that two of your closest friends are in the kitchen with you eating dinner. Let's also assume that all of you are getting along, not fighting or ignoring each other. Together you will form an energetic whole, far more than the sum of the parts. Your auras will interpenetrate.

For the time being, you will have formed a group body.

The phenomenon is familiar, something you have experienced ever since your mother first soothed you to sleep in her arms and along the way the two of you became one. Group body happens all the time (though usually with more withholds than between a baby and mother). The new and fascinating part of group body occurs when you consciously watch it happen.

Even without aura reading, a person can become more aware of group body simply by choosing to become aware. The easiest method is to affirm, "I am part of a group body with the people in this room. I choose to become aware of this now."

Profound though this shift in consciousness may be, however, it is Tater Tots® compared to the magnificent potato salad you will get by adding one more aura reading technique.

That technique comes from connecting to the energy center Katrina Raphaell calls the *soul star*. Located about six inches above the head, its purpose (in my language, not hers) is to wake up a deep spiritual level of identity, each person's I AM essence.

Soul star presents an overview of that person's spiritual being, as if seen from a higher level.

And here's a technique for you to use the soul star to read group body. It prepares you to break through one of the biggest illusions of earth.

Are people really separate, unconnected from each other? It may seem that way now. But from the perspective of celestial consciousness, you'll find it to be a myth.

For this technique you will need both yourself and a group with which you are friendly.

Group Body Awareness

1. Before you join the group, use your primary sensor hand or look in a mirror and use clairvoyance to connect with your own soul star.

2. Set the intention to be aware of group body.

3. Briefly read the soul stars of each member of the whole group (use auravision, touchy sight, empathy, or truth knowledge). As with any subtle perception, don't struggle to get it perfect. Give it a light touch.

4. Know that your awareness is now plugged into group body. You need not focus on soul stars or any other chakra. Allow your awareness to drift and shift; as much information as you can handle will come to you without effort.

5. When you leave the group, intentionally reset your energetic boundaries around yourself and use the centering technique.

With practice, your sessions of group body gazing will bring a strong feeling of connectedness. Your reading will go beyond noticing who is talking, who is leading, at any given moment. Your reading will go beyond telephone awareness and transcend empathy. To consciously enter into group body is something different from all this, a spiritual adventure that unifies you with the entire group.

From that level of identity, you will be the whole circus, three rings and all. At will, you will be able to shift your awareness to any member of the group, much as you now can intentionally shift awareness to your right ear or left foot.

Remember your early experiments with telephone awareness? The level of group body shows you the flow of give and take for everyone. Your earlier insights were probably pretty abstract: George is sending out energy, Martha is taking it in. Now, with an easy shift of awareness, you can go inside either of their selves to experience the energy flow. Maybe George feels pain in the gut. Maybe Martha has a withhold, a secret resentment that short-circuits her power. You will know about it—not necessarily the content, the energy.

For instance, Martha may be partly engaged in the conversation and partly brooding over a golf game she lost today at the country club. Don't expect to know the score, or even that it was a golf loss, but you will know the essence. It's a kind of unity between your identity and that of another person.

Therefore, awareness of group body won't mean being loaded down with specifics. You will simply feel Martha's energy glitch. The form your knowledge takes will depend on your spiritual gifts. Thus, you might tune in empathically on her frustration or the stiffness in the lower part of her right leg (where the experience has been temporarily stored).

Examples can only hint at the richness and fascination of this level of aura reading. If you like the concept of reaching out to others via the Internet, you're going to love this.

Protect Yourself from Evil

What about evil? Subtle perception shows problems, not just prettiness. The prospect of encountering evil has frightened some of my students, and many more have demanded a discussion of this topic for the sake of completeness. So here goes.

What should you do when someone's aura shows evil? You could look at Harry's third eye, for instance, and see black malevolence. Well, note it. Consult your inner dictionary if you have any doubt what it means. File the information for future reference. Then turn your attention away.

The same goes for negative psychic phenomena, such as disembodied spirits, blobs of stress, and ugly thought forms. If subtle perception reveals them to you, say hello and goodbye.

What you put your attention on grows stronger in your life. Especially if you are an empath, don't linger over people who intend harm or are terribly unbalanced. The former don't want your help. The latter may, but are you qualified? Have you even been invited? Don't hang around with sickos unless you have received enough training to know how to proceed effectively (and in a way that keeps you from getting caught up in the stuff), topics outside the scope of this book.

Distancing yourself from evil isn't cowardly. It's smart.

Spiritual cowardice could, in fact, be defined as the belief that evil has the power to harm you. This leads to the need to engage with it in an active struggle.

Another form of cowardice is denial, pretending the evil before your eyes doesn't exist. Face it. To blind yourself to unpleasantness is to dull yourself, psychologically and spiritually. Aura reading can inform you; it clarifies problems that otherwise would show up as vague feelings of anxiety.

**When your perception shows you evil, recognize it.
Then choose to move on.
And know that this sequence in itself is one of the most
powerful spiritual protections in the universe.**

What are other ways to protect yourself? For starters, do your best to stay in balance. Take care of your health. You know the drill: Get plenty of rest, preferably going to bed by 10:00. Avoid alcohol and drugs. Eat moderately. Choose food that agrees with you.

Hard though this plodding sort of discipline may be, the rewards are great. And the next section of this book shows you ways to use your subtle perception to lighten up the chore of keeping in physical balance.

Yet one more way to protect yourself from evil is to choose what is good for you in other aspects of life. In part, this is dealt with in the consumer techniques of this book's final chapter. Subtle perception gives you a more complete view of reality which, in turn, can assist you in choosing real friends, valuable purchases, and the like.

Should evil still be a concern, you can learn extra techniques for grounding your energy, shielding your aura, sending astral entities on their way, and so forth. Ask around until you find a teacher who can show you these things. (My source was The Teaching of the Inner Christ, found in the Bibliography.)

Last, and by no means least, you can always ask God for spiritual protection. In any situation where you feel uncomfortable or scared, remember that the force of good is omnipresent. Every heartfelt prayer receives an answer.

Chapter 5

Read Auras for Better Health

*E*very believer in holistic health knows the key concepts.

- Definition of good health means far more than the absence of symptoms.
- Harmony of body, mind, and spirit are the goal.
- Prevention can eliminate many health problems.
- Responsibility for health and healing belongs to the individual, not doctors.
- Lifestyle choices can make or break health in the long run.

In theory, these concepts about health are profound. Too often the results they produce are disappointing.

Problem is, it takes consciousness to balance spirit, body, and mind. Otherwise, huge discoveries for healing shrink down into gimmicks. Aromatherapy, for instance, can have genuine healing power. But without inspired choice of fragrance, results may last no longer than a spritz of room freshener.

All too often, a believer in holistic medicine expects the "spirit" part of health to be taken care of by daily meditation or prayer. However, spiritual awareness must be applied *along* with each healing technique. Otherwise the technique becomes an empty parody of itself.

Here's where aura reading comes in. Holistic techniques bring deeper results when applied with celestial perception. Fun increases, too, as you'll see. And this chapter doesn't just deal with recognized holistic healing technologies like aromatherapy. You'll also learn how certain everyday activities can become good medicine. These are things you're already doing, like sex, fudge, and rock 'n roll. For starters, have you ever considered the therapeutic effect of kissing babies?

Kissing Babies

Politicians love to kiss babies. The rest of us find it irresistible too, though it won't necessarily win us any votes when the kid's mother is a total stranger. As a new mother, I remember being shocked when passersby would march right up and touch the little miracle that Mitch and I thought belonged to us. No words of introduction, they just touched him, got their blessing and left.

Still, I understood. Especially as an aura reader, I understood. Aside from the obvious sweetness and light in babies, their energy feels like a fountain of youth. And it's BIG.

Aurically speaking, the tiniest baby is a giant.

So the next time a baby comes into view, do yourself a favor. Take the biggest, best look you can, and not just at the obvious cute parts like miniature fingers. Behold the pure, vibrant energy that enfolds a healthy baby like enormous rose petals.

Auric Contact High

Babies' auras may give the quickest contact highs on the planet. Read them whenever you can. These exquisite auras can turn any day into Christmas. Like the Magi at the manger with Jesus, you can witness, adore, and be spiritually lifted.

1. For the clearest experience, catch babies when awake (not as easy as it sounds, since four of their five states of consciousness involve sleep of one sort or another). Do aura bounce, then aura rub. Or find your way in with auravision.

2. Inwardly ask for your aura reading to be enriched through additional subtle senses like emotional empathy, physical empathy, truth knowledge, and emotional touch.

3. What if the child is asleep? True, sleep leaves a baby's aura collapsed like a folded-up umbrella. But look in the child's direction. Look at the person who holds the infant and, if you can, do Step #1, then Step #2. If subtle touch would be too conspicuous and your subtle sight doesn't happen to be working, simply look where the caregiver's aura would be if you could see it and use Step #2.

4. If you have used your primary sensor hand for the reading, finish with an auric seal.

Between mother and baby, you will see the swirling and merging energy exchange of lovers. Without making the trip to the art museum, suddenly you'll find yourself watching masterpieces by Michelangelo, Leonardo da Vinci, and Raphael. Or their equivalent.

Direct auric contact with a wakeful baby brings a spiritual lifting, marked by inner wakefulness and joy that can last for hours. Whether conscious about what they're doing or not, people who steal up to babies for a quick pat are charging themselves up with *darshan*–the contact high you get from a saint.

Believe me, you'll receive even more darshan if you pause your hand at the aura rather than the baby's body. The mothers will like you better, too.

How to Parent an Aura

Rosier delights of parenting notwithstanding, much of a mother's job involves a bizarre sort of health watch. Just as a mom's social personality becomes fragmented, due to keeping one eye on her child during all conversations with others (kind of a perpetual cocktail party without the consolation of drinks), part of a mother's awareness goes on security duty as Health Monitor.

Is Baby Huey too warm, or Toddler Roger too cranky? Could yet one more ear infection be making its nasty presence known? Ugh, is the family about to undergo another togetherness experience that involves the tender sharing of approximately a zillion tissues?

Parenting is doctoring.

Therefore it behooves any parent to learn how to read the little one's aura. Start on a day when your child is delightful: between maladies, awake, and in high spirits. Check out every chakra. Energetically, that is the image of your kid to carry around with you like a wallet photo: your child as a picture of health.

Every day from then on, check the chakras. Just take a glance, as it were. Make this part of your daily routine. For an infant, the most practical method may be a quick aura bounce and seal while changing diapers.

What if one part of your child's body, like the ears, is vulnerable? Be especially sure to read the aura over that part of the physical body. It's worth more than a thousand kid words.

Depending on your child's age, you may be able to get away with a chakra-scan technique especially informative for those with gustatory gift-edness: Sniff the aura over each chakra. On babies, especially, the crown chakra and third eye can transport you into bliss.

Checkups using subtle sight and touch can continue as your child grows older. Incidentally, you will become a role model.

**Teach your child that life includes paying attention
to auras, touching them, talking about them.
Imagine how you would have gained
from having parents who were aura readers.**

One of the biggest surprises during my first years as a mother came after I gave my toddler a session of remote energy healing. As a graduate of advanced Reiki, I had learned techniques to examine Wiggly Boy long distance. While he played with his father downstairs, I sat in my bedroom, scanning his subtle body for physical ailments. Telepathically Matt chatted with me. Meanwhile I sent healing energy where he needed it. Afterwards I ended the session.

Immediately, flesh-and-blood Matty ran into my room. He threw his arms around me for a hug. Then he scampered back downstairs to play with Dad.

Methods like Reiki, Silva Mind Control, and the technique for remote healing in *Flower Essences* (see Bibliography) can increase your skill at healing the aura long distance. They come in handy if your child won't sit still long enough to be worked on.

Learn a method for remote healing if you can. Maybe you won't use it daily. But consider it a worthwhile investment even if you only develop enough skill to prove to yourself you can do it. Validation, even one time, of energy work done long distance is a golden experience of spiritual learning, guaranteed to change forever your acceptance of life's illusions.

High-Vibe Sex

Sex has been described as "the urge to merge." Aurically the partners merge, too. Making love means that you expand your aura to mingle with that of your mate.

And did you know that the mingling continues for several days afterward? That's one compelling reason for partners to demand mutual fidelity. Even if sexually transmitted diseases, especially AIDS, weren't a danger, who would knowingly choose to link to the aura of one's partner's other partner(s)?

Sex can seem mainly physical. Or in the head. Alternatively, it can draw you into a total sharing of energy, including a clearly perceived spiritual high. The choice is yours.

When you open up to the knowledge of auras, eventually it dawns on you that sexual attraction transcends interest in body parts. Energetically you desire a particular partner because your soul finds potential benefit in your blended energies. Similarly, that's why you become desirable to someone else.

Clearly (complicatedly, too) sex involves many motivations besides spiritual linkage. This discussion of auric attraction is not to dismiss the value of dressing attractively or taking a bath. Rather, the auric element matters as much as the more obvious physical enticements.

An energy perspective on real sexiness can be particularly helpful for someone obsessed with looking good. Karen, a recovering bullimic, never thought her body looked sexy enough. She was told, "Stop worrying about your breasts and your thighs. Your soul is what makes you attractive. Either a man will be attracted to your energy or he won't." Realizing this was true, Karen gained a new kind of sexual self-esteem. It was a turning point in her recovery.

Pornography doesn't satisfy because it defines sex in an incomplete and therefore distorted way. Strictly speaking, sexual arousal need only involve one chakra (usually the second or first). Even that one chakra may be partly closed off during a limited act of sexual release.

But the greater the willingness to share with a partner, the fuller the involvement of all the chakras. And the fuller this involvement, the better the orgasm. When you stroll back down memory lane, pausing to consider your most satisfying lovemakings, which chakras were involved? Every one of them can make a vital contribution to your sex life. The table on the following page gives an overview.

Sex for the Whole Chakra System

Component of Positive Sexual Sharing	Symptom of Chakra Imbalance	Corresponding Chakra	
Trusting your partner	Feeling like a piece of meat, not personally acknowledged or involved	#1	Root
Playful physicality, Freedom to express yourself	Inhibition	#2	Lower abdominal
Feeling powerful, strong	Feeling like a victim, you can't get what you want	#3	Solar plexus
Receiving love Giving love	Not receiving love Not giving love	#4	Heart
Communication Telling the truth	Withholds on sharing Lying, faking	#5	Throat
Awareness of the spiritual level of sex Feeling "This is right"	Not aware of the spiritual level of sex Guilt feelings	#6	Third eye
Deep willingness to share energy	Blockage to sharing on a deep level	#7	Crown

Tantra

Lovemaking can be approached as a spiritual path to enlightenment. This is the goal of Tantra, an offshoot of Hinduism that has been practiced for thousands of years. Aurically, Tantra begins every time you open up your chakras to mingle them with a partner. Tantra can be the spiritual study of a lifetime. (You could do worse, right?)

Books devoted to this subject can be a help, and some of the illustrations are a big plus. They may not thrill like the cover of a racy novel but they can deliver interesting information.

But don't wait until you can browse in the Tantra section of your favorite bookstore. Use aura reading right now to introduce yourself and your partner to spiritual sex. Before and after sharing your energies, read your chakras and those of your partner. Your reading can include styles of aura reading that require a high degree of intimacy:

- In the style of The Heart of the Heart technique, hug your partner with one ear positioned to listen to each of the chakras, one at a time. In each position, allow your act of listening to project you into that aspect of your partner's energy field.

- Or tone to each chakra before and after sex.

- Most intimate of all, use subtle smell. Position your nose next to one chakra at a time. Avoid touching the skin, which can be distracting, but otherwise draw as close as you need to take a good whiff. Check with your inner dictionary to interpret the abstract messages you receive.

After these experiments, graduate to the following technique.

Sexual Chakra Connection

If you have already enjoyed the intimacy of intercourse, you're going to love this subtler level of making a connection. Prepare in advance by reading the instructions. You will form a general idea of what to do, which is all you'll need. Anyway, who wants to stop in the heat of passion to turn the page?

1. Inform your partner. Inviting your partner to explore along with you can add to the fun.

2. During foreplay, feel yourself drawing closer to your partner: your senses, your emotions, your total self.

3. While merging, consciously connect chakras. Visualize light or heat at your partner's root chakra, then at your own. Next do your partner's lower abdominal chakra, then your own, and so forth, all the way up the chakras. Don't force yourself to visualize clearly or for a long time, just set the intention to connect.

4. If appropriate, invite your partner to do Step #3 along with you. The synergy will raise vibrations for you both. However, you can have a perfectly good experience if your partner does not choose to pursue this aspect of your being together.

5. When someone is about to climax (your partner or you or both), set the intention to merge your energy fully with your partner. Hold back nothing. Affirm this intention, whether mentally or verbally, with a statement like this: "I call on my Higher Self to fully merge my energy with that of my partner."

6. As part of the afterplay, enjoy an auric treat: stand in front of a mirror with your partner. Look at how you're sparkling with each other's energy. Even those who don't ordinarily see auras very clearly will enjoy this spectacle.

Doing Grace

Maybe you already say grace as a matter of religious principle. Maybe you don't bother, because you grew up with grace as an empty formality. Or maybe the idea of stopping for grace simply doesn't enter your mind.

In any case, aura reading will bring a new perspective.

Amazing Grace

1. Sit down to a meal. If other people are present, it would be a courtesy to give advance notice that you'll be reading auras before and after grace.

2. Place your hands in sensor position above the food on your plate. See, feel, hear, taste, and smell the energy. This is your auric before picture of the food.

3. Keep your hands in sensor position as you say grace, either silently or aloud. Simultaneously, you'll be blasting the food with energy. You may even feel the food's aura change and grow beneath your palms.

4. Repeat Step #2, this time as an auric after picture. Notice the difference?

**Without aura reading, who would have thought
a simple prayer could make such a big,
quick transformation? Many spiritual matters
must be taken purely on faith,
but the effect of grace on food is not one of them,
not for an aura reader.**

Mystery Spice

Imagine a spice you can sprinkle over any food to help your body digest it better. Though you can't buy this spice in a bottle, you can manufacture and apply it directly through your aura. Try this technique the next time you sit down to a meal:

Manufacture Mystery Spice

1. Use your primary sensor hand to feel the energy coming from the food.

2. Cupping both hands, scoop a generous portion of energy out of your solar plexus chakra. Turn your hands over the plate so that you heap this new layer of energy directly onto your food.

3. Repeat Step #1. Notice how your food's energy level has changed?

4. Eat and enjoy.

What you have done is to mix your digestive energies with the food before you eat. Especially if you have food allergies, you'll handle the food better now. Incidentally, don't worry about the energy you scooped out of your solar plexus chakra. It will regenerate in seconds.

Morning Checkup

Sure, consult the Doc when a health problem strikes. But next time, strike back in advance with a pounce of prevention. Aura reading enables you to sneak up on ailments by giving yourself an auric checkup every morning.

Your day's self-exam will take minutes. And you can do it while you brush your teeth, shave, or style your hair.

As you stand before the mirror, blinking sleep from your eyes, shift your vision to your aura.

Some aura readers see colors, others sense a subtle brightness.

Others do their best reading with truth knowledge: address one chakra at a time by looking at it in the mirror. Ask inside, "How are you doing this morning?" Listen inwardly for the answer.

As usual, the trick is to use whichever subtle perception brings you information most easily. Go with the flow and your skill will develop fastest.

A daily checkup first thing in the morning will set you up for a day of using your subtle perception.

The more regularly you do it, the clearer your perception will become and the better you will integrate this aspect of higher consciousness with your everyday life.

Besides that, a morning checkup has the advantage of alerting you to possible health problems right when they first occur—which is when they will be easiest to treat. The rest of the sections in this chapter offer techniques to use subtle energy for healing. Wouldn't it be great if you could stop a slight symptom before it turned into the kind of illness for which you must call a doctor or alternative health practitioner?

Hands-on Chakra Healing

First thing in the morning, don't just lie there stretching. Use the healing energy in your hands to wake up and balance your chakras. Simultaneously you will be developing your subtle sense of touch.

1. Place your left and right hands, in sensor position, directly on your body at the first and second chakra positions, respectively.

2. You can choose to become aware of two different ways your hands work with energy.

   - Receiving. Use your primary sensor hand to receive information. Ask what is going on with each chakra. Listen inwardly for the answer.

   - Giving. Feel energy flow through your alternate sensor hand. Everyone has healing energy to some degree. This laying on of hands will make you more aware of it. Keep your hand in place for a minute or longer. Can you feel the flow of energy energize your chakras?

3. Raise your hands upward 4-6 inches, as if doing Aura Rub. But this time hold your hands still. As in the previous step, direct both hands to receive and give energy, respectively.

4. Decide which style you prefer, hands-on healing or hands-over. Choose one for the rest of this process. Then repeat Step #2 or 3 with chakras 1 and 2, then with 3 and 4, then 5 and 6, 7 and 1. Finish with the auric seal.

Homeopathy

Homeopathy is a natural form of medicine that once was as widely accepted as "regular" allopathic medicine. In America, homeopathy lost its popularity after the American Medical Association won the right to limit official medical training to allopathy. In Europe, though, homeopathy has never gone out of style. An estimated 42% of British doctors refer their patients to homeopathic practitioners.

Today many Americans are thrilled to life about homeopathy. Some remedies have even found their way into supermarkets. Unlike drugs, homeopathic remedies produce no side effects and cost very little. Even better, with some initial training you can prescribe remedies for your family as a form of first aid.

Of special appeal to an aura reader, homeopathy is an energy-based form of medicine. For reasons too technical to detail here, homeopathic remedies are so subtle they have more to do with consciousness than physical properties.

To begin using homeopathy, you can go the route of consultation with a trained homeopathic practitioner. Call the National Center for Homeopathy (703/ 548-7790) for the name of one near you.

Another choice is self-teaching, from books like *Everybody's Guide to Homeopathic Medicines* (see Bibliography). When symptoms of illness first appear, you select the appropriate remedy from a set of many possible choices.

Our household homeopathic pharmacy consists of a 50-remedy kit, a five-year supply whose entire cost was less than one course of the antibiotics it made unnecessary. These kits can be purchased mail order from specialized pharmacies.

Choosing remedies is where homeopathy becomes tricky and aura reading becomes important.

Homeopathy offers remedies for everything from the heartbreak of psoriasis to the grief of divorce. For a cold your reference book may describe 20 sets of symptoms, one for each potential remedy. Your job is to choose the best match. (Misdiagnosed low-strength remedies don't produce side effects. They simply don't work.)

When it comes to remedy choices, aura reading makes your job much easier:

Remedy Finding Technique

1. Look up the ailment in your do-it-yourself homeopathy text. Narrow down your selection to the smallest possible number of remedies.

2. Center yourself.

3. Do an aura bounce and rub, or use visual touch, at the part of the body where the symptoms are worst. You can do this for yourself or a family member. If you're feeling someone else's aura, you may be amazed at how you can identify the exact quality of pain or discomfort.

4. Ask your patient to hold the first remedy bottle (when the patient is yourself, place it in your alternate sensor hand). Feel with your primary sensor hand what happens around the ill person's aura. Check this information with your inner dictionary.

5. Repeat Step #4 with each remedy. The correct choice will make itself clear.

Treats result from this clever trick. First, the remedy is going to help your patient get well, sometimes in a dramatic manner, sometimes more gradually. Second, homeopathic remedies really move around auric energy.

Especially in the case of a high potency remedy, prescribed by a professional homeopathic practitioner, immediate results are amazing.

So before you or a family member take a remedy, position yourself to observe the auric shift. Use auravision or your primary sensor hand. Wow!

Flower Essences

Did you know that, for some people, flower remedies work better than tranquilizers, anti-depressants, and other drugs?

Like their homeopathic cousins, flower and garden essences are subtle healers derived from natural substances. Working on an energy level, they can rebalance the emotions and body. (Of course it's important to consult your health professional before taking remedies. And never discontinue prescription drugs without talking to your doctor.)

One simple introduction to flower essences is to purchase a bottle of Rescue Remedy from your nearest health food store. Then the next time you suffer an injury—physical or emotional—take a few drops as directed on the bottle. Amazing!

Rescue Remedy is a composite of several Bach flower essences, ones that deliver quick comfort. Dozens of individual remedies heal different psychological imbalances. Another superb option is the Perelandra Rose and Garden Essences. (Note: These are available exclusively through Perelandra, see Bibliography.) By now, products like these are big business, with hundreds of choices available.

Test Remedies Aurically

How can you tell which flower remedies to use? The information that comes with the bottle may be minimal. What if you feel bad without knowing why? Depression, minor infection, or major energy shifts may be going on long before you know it. How can your conscious mind figure out what you need most?

Or your conscious mind could even be mistaken. It's hard to see yourself objectively. Pre-aura reading, some of my cherished choices based on descriptions have been dead wrong. The energy didn't fit. Once I paid my chiropractor to break the truth to me, now I do it for myself. You can too.

Several testing methods are available. In *Flower Essences*, author Machaelle Small Wright gives detailed instructions for kinesiological testing. Similar to muscle testing by a chiropractor, the result is in the form of "yes" or "no."

Flashy stuff, this, when you encounter it for the first time. Like dowsing rods and pendulums, methods of kinesiological testing validate the human energy field in ways concrete enough to win over most skeptics.

Simple yes or no answers from kinesiology, though, are really just a good beginning. By contrast, aura testing supplies information that is far more complete and detailed. The following aura reading shortcut enables you to test remedies by the bunch.

Subtle Remedy Discernment

1. Hold your primary sensor hand in front of a group of bottles. If you own a box of assorted remedies, remove the lid. In a store, stand before the display with your primary sensor hand six inches above the bottles. You will scan one row, from the top, at a time.

2. Consciously remind yourself, if necessary, to NOT read the labels. Thus you'll bypass mere ideas about what the remedies do plus any recol-

lections about what you needed last time. Energy field testing will show what you need in the here and now.

3. Moving your hand across the row of remedies, you will feel energy only from those bottles that have something to offer. Most bottles won't. That's why this technique is a shortcut.

4. Go back to each bottle that flagged your attention. Hold it to your solar plexus, using your alternate sensor hand. An aura rub of your third chakra with your free hand will reveal the remedy's effect.

5. Choose the essence that offers you most. Follow the directions on the bottle.

Aromatherapy

Fragrances for aromatherapy can be powerful mood enhancers, consciousness raisers, even healers. Purchase is deceptively simple. Sure, you know what you like.

But what if you like too many fragrances? You can't march out with half the items in the store. Besides you're seeking results beyond a temporarily happy nose. Which aromas will work best for you?

Education is one route. You can study books, read lengthy descriptions. Or—you guessed it—ask your aura. Here's a method that helps you set priorities by using a combination of subtle perception and intuitive knowledge.

Master Technique for Self-Healing

1. Ask your inner dictionary to give you a *priority goal*. Considering all the healing you could request for your entire mind-body-spirit system, what would be most beneficial? Set an intention to receive your priority goal for now.

   - Juanita wants to strengthen her feelings of self-esteem.

   - Ted has digestive pain. More than anything he would like it to stop.

   - Greg feels angry. Calming down is his priority.

   - Elsie's back goes out a lot. She would like to heal the underlying spiritual or psychological cause.

2. Feel your chakras or look at them. Assess which chakra this issue is most connected with—and be prepared for an answer you didn't expect.

For instance, Juanita's problem about "feelings of self-esteem" could really indicate a need for more strength in her power center. She's used to thinking about everything in terms of feelings, so this is the first route by which information can reach her. When Juanita does Step #2, she can discover which chakra to address.

3. Once you have established which chakra needs help most, take it shopping. Hold one aromatherapy product at a time up to the chakra, using your alternate sensor hand; with your primary sensor hand, feel the effect on your chakra. Buy and use the product that produces the desired effect.

The Healing Power of Music

"Music hath charms to soothe a savage breast," said 17th century poet William Congreve. It's still true today. And the trick is finding the music that soothes and suits you best. As an aura reader, you're in a position to understand this from a profound level, a level with the power to heal you, body and soul.

**Music moves energy.
In fact, each musical instrument has
an especially strong effect
on one or more of the chakras.**

Here's how you can find out for yourself. (Incidentally, this technique makes a fantastic party game.)

Aura Music

1. Select several CD's or tapes, each featuring a different kind of instrument, preferably including a solo. If possible, have each of the following ready to play, one at a time:

   - String instruments that can be played with a bow, like violins and cellos

   - String instruments that are plucked, such as harps and guitars

   - Brass instruments, like trumpets

   - Drums

- Flutes or recorders
- Wind instruments played with a reed, such as oboes
- A low-pitched instrument, like bass fiddles, and bassoons
- Any other instrument you especially like

2. Take an auric before picture of each of the main seven chakras. Use toning, primary sensor hand, or auric sight.

3. Play each musical selection for three minutes or longer.

4. Take an auric after picture of each chakra, using the same method you chose for Step #2. What did you notice?

Results reflect more than the consciousness of the composer and musicians, though these are naturally factors. Instruments themselves speak to the chakras. Effects could be soothing or enlivening, depending on the style and tempo of the music.

**Whatever else music may do, music is medicine.
Prescribe it according to chakra.**

For instance, have you ever had to drive a long distance, fighting off sleep at the wheel, and no coffee available for miles to come? So you would turn on the loudest rock 'n roll you could find to get yourself through. You knew it worked, but why?

The energy explanation is that rock music (and to a greater extent, rap music) arouses the primal energy of the second chakra. No wonder it has such an appeal for adolescents, with their incredible hormonic convergence.

So next time some teen with blaring boom box in hand sends you screaming for cover, peek at the poor kid's lower abdominal chakra. Now that's energy!

Affirmations through All Your Senses

Millions of people find magic in statements like "I like myself," "I am perfect health," and "Let go and let God." It's well known that affirmations are positive statements, spoken aloud, and chosen to improve the quality of life. Less known: these life-transforming, health-bringing words become far more effective when you combine them with aura reading.

The techniques that follow have proven their worth for me and my students. Whether you're a veteran affirmer or a novice, start with this:

Words of Power

"Sticks and stones may break my bones but words will never hurt me." Says who? This technique shows the impact of words on your energy.

1. Take an auric before picture of your third chakra. Bounce and rub with your primary sensor hand, watch your chakra in the mirror, or tone. It's important to find language for this reading. (If no words jump out at you, consult your inner dictionary.)

2. Speak this affirmation: "I am powerful."

3. Repeat Step #1. What did this affirmation do to your power energy?

4. Speak this statement out loud: "I am a victim."

5. Repeat Step #1. (Immediately afterward say "Cancel" to wipe out negative subconscious programming from the previous statement.)

6. Speak this affirmation: "I am powerful because I am a good person."

7. Repeat Step #1.

Read Your Subconscious through Your Aura

To explain how affirmations work, teachers usually make mysterious reference to your subconscious mind and how its beliefs create conditions related to behavior, health, and happiness. But hold on!

**Your subconscious mind shows in your aura.
So you can get immediate feedback
on the subconscious impact of any words you say
by testing your reaction on the level of energy.**

This gives you the ability to use affirmations like a master. For instance, no more wasting time with an affirmation you don't need. Try out one power statement after another, testing your third chakra afterwards. Some statements will help, others may actually hinder.

Your aura will show you that some popular affirmations do absolutely nothing for you, personally. Ever hear of this one? "Every day, in every way, I am getting better and better."

Generations ago, Emile Coué's "Formula for Self-Cure Through Faith" swept the nation. In its day it worked wonders, and the idea certainly sounds appealing. But having tried it out, with all respect to the memory of Mr. Coué, I must say it did zilch for me.

And that brings up a big problem with affirmations: time management. Even if a whole bunch of affirmations sound good, how many are worth your while? More than three per day are probably too many—unless you plan to get into affirmations full time.

Why theorize about what your subconscious needs to hear the most? You can ask directly, as demonstrated in the following technique:

Affirmation Effectiveness Test

1. Check out Chakras #1-6 with your primary sensor hand or auravision. (Why not check out Chakra #7? As discussed previously, it's already quite perfect.)

2. Feel which chakra needs attention most. Choose one to be the focus of your affirmations for the next week.

3. Experiment with different positive statements directed towards that particular chakra. Find these affirmations in books or make them up yourself. For example, here are some helpful declarations for the root chakra:

   - "It is safe to be me."
   - "I am confident about every aspect of my life."
   - "I release all fear of not having enough money. I always have plenty of money because God is the source of my supply."

4. Check in with your chakra after saying each affirmation. Keep observing for a full minute because an especially powerful affirmation can seem to have a depressing effect for the first few seconds, as it neutralizes old fears. This done, the aura bounces back even stronger than before you spoke the affirmation.

   When you have found an especially effective combination of words, or used a technique that succeeds brilliantly, you may notice an *auric flare*. This burst of light around one or more chakras signals that you have dramatically upgraded your energy.

5. Choose the three affirmations that make your chosen chakra the strongest.

Love or Lying?

One of the bigger points of controversy among affirmation users concerns the extent to which it is advisable to stretch the truth. Currently you weigh 160 pounds, let's say. Should you try to reach your ideal weight by affirming, "I make the lifestyle choices that bring my weight to a healthy 120 pounds"? That's quite a shrink. Will it work?

Some experts say you'd have better results from using a more realistic figure, affirming a loss of five pounds at a time. Which choice is right for you?

The controversy boils down to this: Should you tell your subconscious a little white lie? Even if you don't believe the affirmation, maybe your subconscious will fall for it and create a reality to match. Stretching credibility can thus be seen as an act of love. Besides, why limit the reality of your subconscious mind? Truth is relative.

Another view doesn't agree that lying to oneself can make life better, at least for long.

Aura reading bypasses the entire debate. Find out how *your* subconscious reacts on a case-by-case basis.

Your chakras know if an affirmation feels like an inspiration or a lie.

Once you select an affirmation to work with, why not test it?

Affirmation Believability Test

1. Position your hand or eyes to examine your throat chakra. Read the energy.

2. Speak out your affirmation.

3. Read the energy again. What happened?

If the results show discomfort in your throat chakra, the affirmation flunks. Don't try to talk your brain into liking something your speech center hates. As you learned in an earlier chapter, throat chakras aren't stupid. They don't like "I don't know" and they don't like repeating words that feel wrong.

Many devoted affirmers have clogged their throats so badly, they come across as phony all the time, not only during their sessions of self-talk. So no matter how tempted you may be to stretch the truth beyond what your subconscious finds believable, don't. Affirm a level of truth that an open throat chakra can live with.

Affirm with Celestial Power

Whew, your affirmation has passed all tests. Now what? Bypass boring affirmation techniques of plain repetition. Instead try the following methods, effective because they activate one or more gifts of celestial perception. The closer you are to the seed level of senses when you affirm, the more powerfully you will manifest your heart's desire.

Connect with the Energy of the Elements

Poets, you're going to love these ways to use your words of truth.

1. Write down the words of your affirmation and read them by candlelight.

2. Sing your affirmation while you run water through your fingers.

3. Hurl your words into a howling wind as it tosses your hair.

4. Stand outside barefoot. Feel your feet tap into the richness of the soil as though they were roots. Speak your affirmation. Feel how your words, too, become grounded into the earth.

Search for Spiritual Treasure

Discovering spiritual treasure means finding the special excellence in something or someone. Why not go on a treasure hunt where you are right now?

1. Examine what is around you as though visiting for the first time. Soon as you find something beautiful, focus on it while you speak your affirmation one time.

2. Find another color, shape, texture, sound, or smell that appeals to you as beautiful. Pay attention to it while you speak your affirmation one time. Beauty, like newness, brings power to your words of healing.

3. Repeat the previous step again and again, so long as you're having fun.

As James Redfield pointed out in *The Celestine Prophecy*, beauty is just a shorthand term for a perception that helps your awareness shift to a higher vibration. I would add, the higher the vibration, the subtler your perception. Affirmations with higher awareness and subtler perception bring stronger results.

Affirmations Made Catchy

1. Any time that a song or commercial jingle runs through your head, rename that tune. Use the familiar melody as backup music for an affirmation. Another possibility is to invent your own catchy tune.

   For example, combine "I accept myself" with a simple melody like "Happy Birthday to You." Sing: "I accept myself. I accept myself. I accept myself. I accept myself."

2. After you sing, bring your subtle hearing into play. Sing the affirmation mentally, chanting slower and softer each time, until it fades into silence.

   For example, sing this now in the softest of mental whispers: "I accept myself. I accept myself. I accept myself. I accept myself."

Hug with Words

The deeper your emotional touch while you affirm, the more profound your results.

1. Hug a stuffed animal or favorite pillow. Become aware of the emotion generated. Speak your affirmation directly into that emotion.

2. Hug a tree. What emotion do you notice? Whisper or chant your words while you focus on that emotion.

3. Choose a good friend to experiment with you. Decide on an affirmation that both of you would like to use. (When hugging under other circumstances, close friends might tell each other, "I love you." A powerful related affirmation for you to share here is "I love *myself*.") Hug your friend. Together, chant the affirmation three times or more.

Welcome to God's Country

1. Everyone has a favorite landscape, be it mountain, ocean, desert, or forest. Choose one now to go to, through imagination, while you affirm.

2. Take yourself to that very place. Pretend you're standing there or look at a photo of the landscape. Otherwise travel there, in imagination, with eyes closed. Have you ever tried travel by listening to a tape of nature sounds?

   How about bringing your favorite landscape to you? Keep a souvenir in your bedroom, such as a jar of beach sand that you can open up and touch. The more concrete your contact the better. If possible, touch something from your landscape, watch it, or listen to the sounds you can make with it.

3. All the while you "travel" to your favorite landscape, affirm out loud.

Texturized Affirmations

1. Dedicate a session of powerful speech to textures. Then go on a texture hunt.

2. Touch the furniture, the floor. Feel items in the room where you are right now (materials like glass, metal, cloth) until you find something that appeals to you.

3. Repeat your affirmation as you rub your fingers back and forth to intensify your experience of the texture you've chosen.

4. The instant you tire of one texture, find another. Resume affirming.

5. Continue until you feel fulfilled. Much as you might know you have eaten enough of a delicious meal, eventually you will have had your fill of touching. Immediately stop touching and affirming. Know that your session has served its purpose.

Say It with Flowers

If you thought you loved flowers before, wow! Inspired by the spiritual perfection of flowers, I've developed a bouquet of affirmation techniques. From Step #2 on, each item can be explored as a separate technique. Or you can do the steps in sequence to form one super-powerful flower technique.

1. To start, select a goal and the words to match it. For instance, you might set the goal to heal your heart chakra; your affirmation statement(s) might be: "I am lucky at love. All the love I give returns to me sevenfold."

   With the following steps you will direct your words to one flower and one sense at a time. (Only one flower available? Treat each petal as a separate flower.)

2. With your first flower use subtle touch to caress its petals. Affirm as you revel in the silky tenderness. Then bring your primary sensor hand out to the aura and caress again. Affirm some more.

3. With the next flower, use analytical awareness to appreciate the exquisite structure of the plant. Each time you notice a nuance, speak your affirmation. You'll be connecting to the creativity and intelligence of the plant's design, a superb way to bring more of these qualities into your life.

4. With the next flower, use gustatory giftedness. Smell the flower's fragrance, enjoying the many layers of experience that may reveal themselves. These subtle layers may be too abstract for words to describe them. But you can use the words of your affirmation to match each level of subtlety. Set the intention that each speaking will enliven the level of fragrance you experience with subtle smell and taste. Then take a deep breath, smell, let your awareness settle on a level of fragrance and speak your affirmation.

   This affirmation technique may be difficult at first, but it's powerful! It's also an excellent way to improve your experience of gustatory giftedness.

5. With the next flower, use physical empathy. Set the intention to feel, as if within your own body, how the consciousness of the flower expresses through its structure. Sound difficult? Too abstract? Then turn this technique into a means of developing your physical empathy.

   Touch or look at the flower and say, as a set of affirmations, "I am developing clear physical empathy. The consciousness of this flower expresses through its physical structure. I am aware of this now. And, further, I temporarily duplicate this pattern within my own physical body. I experience this fully now."

Chapter 6

Save Money with the Aura Advantage

hoever would have thought that subtle perception could help a person save money? Well, aura reading gives you an advantage for buying quality which, as everyone knows, saves money in the long run. You'll see deeper than labels and claims to gauge a product's real effect on your energy.

Amazing! Subtle perception can be amazing. Imagine tasting apples aurically to tell if they're crisp inside. How about predicting what a new brand of shampoo will do for your hair!

Even items that don't touch your physical body can have an effect on your aura. Increasingly, we're consumers of information. Be smart by checking out in advance the energy effects of books, tapes, even seminars. This chapter will show you how to avoid expensive mistakes. All it takes is a few moments of quiet research before you surrender your money.

Another aspect of consumerism is (or should be) fully enjoying what you purchase. I know you'll get a kick out of techniques like the one for reading auras while you watch TV.

Best of all, the techniques in this chapter are just a beginning. Once you get started, you'll discover plenty of new ones that fit with your lifestyle. Let's begin with one of vital importance to those of us whose eyes light up at the thought of FREE FOOD.

Free Food

Superstores and warehouses promise us bargains these days, but the best discount of all comes from shopping with less waste. What if you could add up the money you've squandered on produce that turned out to be sour, bitter, over-ripe, mushy, or tasteless? Cut down on those shopping mistakes, aura reader, and use the savings to buy yourself the equivalent of free food.

If you use your subtle senses with skill you never need buy another package of cheese that's too strong for your taste, never need make the disconcerting discovery that an expensive little juice box has less going for it energetically than a glass of tap water.

Give yourself a discount: Consult your subtle perception every time you shop. Not only will you save money but it's fascinating to explore how subtle perception lets you taste food and feel its texture long before you cut into it.

The conventional wisdom for selecting food remains helpful, of course. Labels are indispensable for processed foods, especially when you've schooled yourself about the more popular tricks to deceive consumers, like including many variants on sucrose to order to avoid labeling the number one ingredient truthfully as sugar.

Next time you buy a condiment, a prepared soup, anything with a label, take auric before-and-after pictures.

How Alive Is This Food Anyway?

1. Select the product you plan to test.

2. Take an auric before picture of your solar plexus chakra. Use toning, primary sensor hand, or auravision.

3. Hold the test product against your side, using your alternate sensor hand.

4. Take an auric after picture of your solar plexus chakra, using the same method you chose for Step #2.

As you'll see, competing products do have more to compare than price. Or the manufacturer's claims.

Produce Results

Whenever possible, don't you prefer to buy ingredients without packaging of any sort? It's easiest to learn about food when you have a chance to poke it directly, to squeeze and sniff and make direct contact. And it's fun to try every tip cooking experts offer for selecting quality.

Still, even the best tips for inspecting food by direct handling fall short in one respect. The food knows itself best. For the most reliable information, let the food talk to you by means of its aura.

Veggies and fruits have especially strong auras. Anything with consciousness has an aura.

One of the main reasons we eat any kind of food is to be nurtured by its consciousness.

The fresher the food when you buy it, the more consciousness remains.

Petrified overcooked string beans, sloshing around for months in a can of brine, won't exactly scintillate. But who would, under the circumstances? When you aurically interview beans, you'll get a snappier response from one alive enough to snap. Here's how I converse with an eggplant, an avocado, or (trickiest of all) a watermelon:

Aura Test Produce

1. Hold the food in your alternate sensor hand (or use that hand to balance the food against your torso, if the item of food is too large for one hand to support).

2. Use your primary sensor hand to examine the food with an aura bounce, then an aura rub. Or look at the food straight in the aura.

3. Ask the interviewee: "Show me how you taste." or "Show me your texture."

4. Zowie, there's the answer ... beneath your hand, before your eyes ... a flavor/texture résumé ... gladly given and totally true.

One caution: Don't expect perfect results the first time you try this technique, but do expect that your development of skill will be cumulative. From the first day you grocery shop as an aura reader, you will say goodbye to meaningless, routine shopping, essentially the same week after week. Starting now, you will school yourself with every shopping trip, moving towards a Ph.D. in Shopping with Celestial Perception.

Along the way, will you make an occasional shopping mistake? Sure. But, significantly, most mistakes will happen simply because you forgot to apply your skills, not because you used them wrong. Thus, mistakes can prod you to develop the habit of remembering. Whenever you go shopping bring along your subtle senses.

No More Dud Flowers

You buy an exotic houseplant from the neighborhood florist or a bunch of carnations from a street vendor. The things look great ... until you bring them home.

Who hasn't suffered from botanical letdown? As an aura reader you can tell when flowers are droopy before they physically drop. The reason is interesting. The energy aspect of a living plant or animal is one step ahead of its physical outpicturing. Therefore you can feel problems before they show up.

An extreme example of this comes from a story about the legendary psychic Edgar Cayce. Cayce was disturbed when he encountered a man who showed no auric energy at all. Sure enough, within 24 hours the man was dead.

Similarly, with flowers, aura reading shows both life and the lack of it. Conveniently you need no technical knowledge of horticulture. Here's what you do need:

Gardener's Basic Aura Technique

1. Place your primary sensor hand a few inches above the flower.

2. Bounce the energy, then rub it.

Aside from the diagnostic benefit, aura reading will also enable you to smell flowers by hand. This is an inconspicuous way to enjoy their fragrance and energy boost without making a spectacle of yourself.

Instead of begging permission to sniff, just let your sensor hand linger over the air a few inches above the blossoms.

Believe me, healthy flowers will give you their best. And they'll still have plenty of fragrance left for the paying clientele.

> **A flower's perfume is a translation
> of its essence energy into the sense of smell.
> Similarly, the flower's visual form
> translates its essence energy into the sense of sight.**

Regarding both facets, form and fragrance, flowers generally do a far better job than people at dressing themselves. They express themselves perfectly, nothing unnecessary added, nothing left out.

For that reason, every budding aura reader should stop to smell the flowers. It is an education to read an aura of such simple perfection. And every time you consciously compare subtle perception with physical scent and shape, you take a mystic's master class in synesthesia.

As for the plants for which you must pay, here too aura reading will be worth its weight in gold. Not only will you avoid buying flowers that turn your fanciest vase into a small ceramic hospital. Now you can flower shop with confidence. Like a honey bee, you'll go straight for the plants with life.

The Wisdom of Trees

A related way to learn from larger plants is similar (though hardly inconspicuous). Have you tried hugging trees? Pick out one you like, wrap your arms around it and touch your third eye to the bark. Even a non-aura reader can usually feel an energy boost. With open intuition, you will feel the tree's presence enfold you, complete with a major blast of auric power.

While you're at it, you can also ask the tree if it has something to teach you spiritually. Make your request in the language of thought, rather than words. Then go within, as though reading your inner dictionary, to receive an answer. (Incidentally, this simple process is good telepathy practice.)

Consult trees for information? Why not? That's just one step beyond finding them an inspiration, which you undoubtedly do already.

Some clairvoyants enjoy watching how these generous energy movers give to everyone who walks past. When you hug or ask they give even more, as your subtle senses will show you. Tree hugging works not only if you're clairvoyant but if you have woken up gifts for clairsentience, clairaudience, gustatory giftedness, truth knowledge, physical and emotional empathy. Wow! To me, tree hugging ranks near the top of the list of Life's Glorious Freebies.

Let Your Plants Talk Back to You

The best gardeners admit they talk to their plants, but aura readers go one better. They can listen.

In the last section you learned how to eavesdrop on a flower's energy field, an approach you can use to avoid buying half-dead houseplants. But what do you do when the beauty you brought home droops several months later?

Gardener's Technique for Clairsentients

1. Rub the plant's aura.

2. Hold still and ask the plant, "What do you need?"

3. Truth knowledge may come directly to you through your outstretched hand. Otherwise consult your inner dictionary while your hand still connects you directly to the plant's energy field.

Alternatively, if you're more clairvoyant than clairsentient, here's a method for you:

Gardener's Technique for Clairvoyants

1. Center yourself.
2. Ask your Higher Self to show the level of the plant's aura which can help you heal it.
3. Open your eyes. Notice what you see around the plant, directly or peripherally. If you need more information, consult your inner dictionary.

Whether you look or touch, the trick is to stay open and receptive. If a thought flashes in your mind, don't dismiss it. You have probably received information from that plant or its *deva* (DAY-vah). For more about devas, the nature spirits that act like plants' guardian angels, read about or visit Findhorn, a Miracle Gro® of a community in Scotland, or Machaelle Small Wright's Perelandra in West Virginia.

Evaluate whatever information you receive about plants in the light of common sense; act on it if the idea seems practical.

Possibly you will have a perception without a thought, for instance a texture or color. What does that mean? Center yourself and consult your inner dictionary.

The more technical your knowledge about soil, plant nutrients, pests, and so forth, the more technical an answer you will be capable of receiving. After all, you wouldn't expect to receive a long list of instructions in Swahili if you couldn't speak enough of the language to say "hello." Often, though, the needs of a plant will not be as complex as you might imagine.

"Help" said Paula. "My flowering plant used to bloom so beautifully. Now it won't make flowers any more.

"It's barely alive," she complained. "And I've moved it around the room, changed the watering schedule, measured out doses of plant food. Nothing seems to do the trick."

What would the plant's aura tell me? First I bounced my hand against it: very low energy. "Listless" was the word that came to mind. I moved my hand inside the aura, which was so small I couldn't avoid brushing against the physical plant; still I focused on the aura. "What's the matter?" I asked.

"I'm lonely," it said. "Put me with other plants."

"Paula," I asked. "Could you move a plant in here to keep this one company?"

She moved several. Within weeks a profusion of new flowers bloomed on the formerly barren plant.

Only years later, reflecting on the experience, did I realize a deeper significance. All living beings are connected, responding to each other on subtle levels. In particular, it's common for plants, animals, and young children to express problems that adults suppress. The plant in Paula's bedroom had taken on some of her loneliness. Both of them needed companionship.

As you open up your sensitivity to plants' auras, seldom will you find sadness. Healthy plants are an inspiration. They radiate joy, nurturing, and exuberance—qualities that can be contagious for the aura reader.

Don't Turn People Away, Turn up the Energy

We've all been there: the deeply dowdy blind date, the boring club meeting, the Thanksgiving that feels more like "Torturegiving." On top of the overall lack of enjoyment, sometimes you have to spend money to be with people in situations like these. Dubious privilege, isn't it?

And even if you don't have to pay financially, your time is worth money. Therefore a wise consumer won't settle for social occasions that seem like a waste. Do something about it. After all you are an aura reader now.

Did you know that any strong emotion raises your energy level? Boredom, irritation, intense dislike— the worse they feel, the more energy they pump into your mind-body system. The big question is, what will you do with it?

Commonly, ways of handling negative energy involve creative squelching techniques. Denial is popular. Stuffing emotions along with large amounts of food, either during or after the occasion—that's tempting. Fidgeting brings a less caloric form of relief, though it exposes your discomfort.

How about the time hallowed method of Mental Running Commentary? (Example: "There goes Uncle Gus again with his disgusting Name Dropping Routine. Whoopee. Oh, now he's playing Nobody Ever Appreciates Me, etc.")

Useful and ingenious though these coping behaviors may be, ultimately they are wasteful. Negative energy still is energy, extra nerve juice. You can feed on it. When you choose to positively revel in your uncomfortable feelings, that large amount of energy can enrich you regardless of the emotion first attached to it. Should you combine that emotional energy with aura reading, you really increase the energy benefits. Here's how:

Handling Annoying People

1. Be aware of your negative feelings, rather than trying to deny them. Unless you're in danger, don't run. For future reference, it's fair to decide to never repeat the visit! But since you're here now, stay a while. Your commitment to staying, in itself, will escalate the energy. And, as long as you're staying, ground yourself.

2. Intensify the energy even more: silently pray for balance in the situation. Ask to have the intensity flow through you in a positive way.

3. Read the aura of the person who has been driving you up the wall. Start with the root chakra and work your way up.

4. Combine detached observation with a personal commitment to learning. When you see a chakra that seems especially unaligned or conflicted, that can solve the mystery of why you feel so uncomfortable. Insight will bring relief and, perhaps, compassion for the person so drastically out of whack.

5. For even better results, go on to check your corresponding chakra. Hear an unexpected shrillness in your voice? Maybe you caught it from Aunt Brittany. And Uncle Julius' deadened power chakra may have unconsciously set off an empathic depression. Recognize the stuff originating from others. Send it on its way by saying inwardly: "All that does not belong to me, leave immediately."

6. For the rest of your visit, continue to monitor the energy patterns, using the technique for telephone awareness.

When you try this experiment, you may be surprised that you can move so much emotion without having to become involved psychologically. You feel the energy. Read it. Shift it. No fuss or muss; don't bother with in-depth psychological analysis. Awareness, all by itself, can move energy.

Master riding the energy. In this case mastery means that you will leave the encounter with your own aura intact, maybe stronger than ever. Outwardly, others may marvel as you tame the social equivalent of a bucking bronco. Inwardly you'll feel like a rodeo winner.

Watch How Movie Stars Shine

Next time you buy a movie ticket, remember that it entitles you to watch auras, the most dazzling cinematography of all. And there's nothing like a big screen plus big stars for spectacular viewing.

Great physical looks are expected from these performers, strong personalities, and technical skill. Maybe you follow the latest gossip about your favorites. But another aspect is far more fascinating:

The most closely held secret about stars of the stage and screen (maybe the only secret) is what amazing auras they have. The stars with careers that last are spectacular energy movers.

Take Robin Williams, for instance. Even to the casual observer, he is clearly not from this planet. (Imagine what earth life would be if everyone had such a fluid, transformative intelligence!) Next time you see him, inspire yourself by reading the energy around his head.

You prefer sex symbols? Stare squarely at their scintillating second chakras. If you liked watching Elvis dance before, you've got to find one of his old movies now. Zoom in on that gyrating aura. And whichever performer you consider the sexiest star today, you're sure to enjoy him or her more when you watch the second chakra.

Love those close-up kissing scenes? You ain't seen nothing yet. Auras show you something far more intense and intimate. Simply set the intention to see what chakras can show you about sexuality.

Third chakras offer a uniquely interesting set of information for aura watchers. Professional performers may be trained to hide their stage fright, but it shows here, even if well hidden otherwise. Next time you see a live show, observe how actors make their entrances. Aim your subtle sight directly at the solar plexus. It's refreshing to see nervousness transmute during the course of a performance.

On film you won't see nervousness. But the big and small screens show plenty of other fascinating power center stuff.

For instance, TV can treat you to an exquisitely sweet, serene third chakra; it belongs to the man whose program has given children a surrogate Dad for generations, Fred Rogers.

Strong third chakras, whether serene or just plain confident, can give you a contact high. And speaking of therapeutic chakras, anyone with throat chakra blockage has got to watch celebrity throats. Singers often have magnificent throat chakras. So do uninhibited actors. Whoopi Goldberg's first name, for instance, is a name-and-form match to her fifth chakra energy.

Heart chakras, during dramatic scenes, reveal how deeply an actor feels the role. Subtle perception brings a new perspective: Who goes beyond looking the part and reacts all the way to the chakras?

If you've wondered why Meryl Streep is considered one of the greatest actresses ever, watch her auric shifts. Most impressively, I've seen her age her aura by a good 30 years. Frail elderly people show a unique insecurity in their auras, especially the root chakra. Fear of falling, of bones that will break, the suffering of chronic pain—it shows. When Streep brought that quality to her aura in one scene of "The Bridges of Madison County," she won my Oscar.

Some performers have highly distinctive auric patterns all around. John Wayne, for instance, had rock-solid chakras whose toughness intensified as he aged. Candice Bergen's performance as rigid, controlling Murphy Brown contrasts deliciously with her quicksilver energy.

My final tip for star gazing is to use aura reading in the cases where you think a performer really stinks. Someone you consider to be highly overrated may turn out to be spectacularly talented—as an energy mover. For instance, if you ever have a chance to see footage of the legendary musical comedy star Ethel Merman, put in earplugs if you must, and prepare for an earthquake. Your aura is about to receive a shakeup. Sudden, intense, and sublime.

Judy Garland was also fascinating on the level of energy. During her prolific early career, her chakras opened right up when she sang, pouring out energy like a typical Hollywood star. During her later years, however, came Garland's truly remarkable performances, aurically speaking. Not only did Garland look tormented; the poor woman's energy field was a wreck. For her to sing through those chakras was a soul-stirring expression of human courage.

Whatever your focus, aura watching will transform your appreciation of all performing artists. The greatest show on earth? It's got to be energy.

Really See that CD

Nearly all music stores allow you to listen as long as you like to a pre-selected CD. But sometimes you don't have the time. The store is crowded. The list of your Saturday errands looms long. So you wind up making a choice based on looking at the packaging, recollections of a review, hearing just a sound bite. It's a gamble.

Why not improve your odds? You guessed it. Take a deeper look. With aura reading, your fingers can do the waltzing.

Preview Music with Auras, Not Just Sound Bites

1. Pick up the compact disc or tape whose purchase you're considering.

2. Center yourself. Put your primary sensor hand six inches away from the tape. Get a feel for the energy coming out of the package.

3. With your alternate sensor hand, place the CD against your solar plexus. Use your primary sensor hand to feel the impact on your fourth chakra, then your third. This will inform you of the overall feeling the music will leave with you, plus your probable gut reaction.

Skeptical? Continue the process of exploration in the privacy of your home. Even better, invite some friends to join you. Ask each one to bring along a recording, then combine a *loud music meditation* with some subtle sensing.

Loud Music, Subtle Sensing

Why do a loud music meditation? The louder the sound, the more the energy of the music blends into each person's aura (which is why music you dislike when soft becomes violently obnoxious when loud). With a Loud Music Meditation you combine this effect with your intent to learn how that music changes your energy. To follow up, go beyond speculation. Aura reading is the perfect follow-up for show and tell.

Loud Music, Subtle Sensing

1. Place all the recordings in a grab bag. Pick one at random. Transfer it to a paper bag.

2. Let each guest try Steps #2 and 3 of the previous technique. Encourage everyone to share impressions out loud. What if your guests haven't learned how to read auras yet and you're not up to giving a lesson? Invite guests to simply hold each disc and give a general impression of its energy. (Technically, this is a simple form of *psychometry*, the art of sensing energy by holding an object. Most of us are naturals at psychometry if we'll just give it a try.)

3. Remove the disc from the bag. Show everyone what it is.

4. Allow the disc to move energy by doing a loud music meditation: Everyone sprawls out on the floor, with pillows optional. Play the music at the loudest volume that is comfortable for all group members.

   Encourage everyone to give feedback about volume. For those with sensitive ears, excessive loudness is a form of torture. For everyone, sensitive or not, excessive loudness causes hearing loss that is irreversible and cumulative.

5. Let the music wash over your guests until the disc is over—or someone screams, "! @ ! ! • # • • *STOP* • • # • ! ! @ !"

6. Back at the group, now that the music has had its effect, invite each guest to read his or her aura, sharing this information with the group.

   For guests who have not learned to read auras yet, simply ask, "How did the music make you feel?" (A side benefit of this approach is that you, the aura reader, will be able to silently compare the kind of information this method yields to your data from aura reading. Often when people are invited to express feelings, they wind up psychologizing in a rambling manner. By contrast, aura reading gives here-and-now information that is far more specific.)

7. Optional: Repeat Steps #2-6 with a different disc pulled from the grab bag.

Eavesdrop on Subliminals

One musical purchase is in a class all by itself, the subliminal tapes where the music comes as a bland background noise and your real purchase can't be heard at all. Affirmations, piped in at a level heard only by your subconscious mind, are designed to reprogram your thinking in a more positive direction. The purpose of a subliminal tape can be general or specific: optimism, prosperity, quit smoking, lose weight.

Have you ever tried one of these tapes? I have found some to be very helpful. But buying them must be the biggest consumer act of faith ever.

For starters, how to judge value? A manufacturer will claim to have the best experts, the largest number of affirmations, or the most sophisticated recording devices. Maybe these factors matter, maybe they don't. What is the real difference between a tape that costs $35 and one that costs $10?

Second, you must take on faith the tape's choice of affirmations. Since your conscious mind won't hear a word, you have no way to screen out messages that are inappropriate for you. What if the tape's 10,000 sentences include 200 you would never consciously choose to swallow?

For instance, an outdated weightloss tape might say: "Pasta and bread are fattening. I hate all starchy foods." By repeating such messages on a daily basis, you might miss out on major health benefits; yesterday's despised starches are today's acclaimed sources of complex carbohydrates.

And what if the tape's authors include some statements that could, inadvertently, be dangerous? "Every day I become thinner than the day before." "Just the thought of overeating makes me feel sick." For the tape's writers, these statements seem like smart ways to avoid excess food. But for you, the programming might trigger an eating disorder.

How can you know what's in your tape? Have you ever found a subliminal packaged with a list of the enclosed affirmations? Very funny. Supposedly that would make the tape less effective.

Aura reading enables you to get around all these roadblocks to buying subliminals. When you consider buying a tape, listen energetically. Although you won't be able to snoop for specific affirmations like "Every day I become thinner," you can eavesdrop on the tape's overall content by hearing how it affects your energy. Besides that, the tape itself has energy—the quality comes from the consciousness of its writers and performers.

Aurically Preview Subliminals

1. Pick up a subliminal tape that seems appealing.

2. Center yourself.

3. Use your alternate sensor hand to place the tape at your waist. With your primary sensor hand, feel the impact on your solar plexus chakra. Do an aura bounce, then rub, to learn exactly what this tape does to your sense of personal power.

4. Now place the tape directly on the crease where one of your legs comes out of the hip joint. With your primary sensor hand, feel the impact on your root chakra. Do an aura bounce, then rub, to learn the impact on your sense of security. Do the affirmations make you feel safe or threatened?

If you discover that one of your chakras doesn't like the tape, pay attention. Forget the promises, the packaging. This tape is not good for you. Buy a different tape, one that perks up your chakras or soothes them.

Beyond the Looks of Books

How do most people choose books? They inspect the cover, jacket blurb, first few pages, last few paragraphs. But there's a better way, faster and more reliable.

Be an intuitive bookworm. Get inside the energy and start chewing.

Otherwise you, the consumer, are at a disadvantage. Editors know how people choose books. (Amazing! And you thought your browsing shortcuts were unique.)

Here's one example of how major publishers use a sophisticated approach, even for designing books that look junky. Research has shown that the best jacket color to move books is red. Beyond that, consider the effects of two different shades of red. Tomato red, with a yellowish undertone, is preferred by men. Women favor red with a bluish undertone. Depending on the target audience for the book, guess what the shade of red will be.

Pretty sneaky, huh?

So you may be manipulated by very superficial means into choosing a book to purchase. After you bring it home, the book may not deliver what the title promised. Or maybe the problem is that the book reflects the author's personality, one you find increasingly incompatible with your own. Even a free book from the library involves a precious investment. Your time.

That's why it pays to aura test a new book. The overall energy will tell you how compatible the book's vibes really are.

Reading Books for Energy

1. Select one book at a time for testing.

2. Center yourself.

3. Hold the book up to your side, using your alternate sensor hand. "Energetically, what is this book going to offer me?" Ask this, then check out the effects on your most appropriate chakra, such as:

   - First chakra for thrillers and detective stories.
   - Second chakra for romances.
   - Third chakra for volumes on politics or history, historical novels, and cookbooks.
   - Fourth chakra for biographies.
   - Fifth chakra for how-to's on communication.
   - Sixth chakra for books on psychology, religion, and metaphysics.

The wrong book, regardless of content, attempts to bring your mind to a place where you don't want to go. But the right book can lead you to places no other medium can reach. Reading can become a powerful meditation, moving your consciousness to the plane from which the author wrote.

Buying Stuff

By now you're getting the picture. Everything worth buying should be energy checked. All it takes is a little time, a little attention. Common sense is a consumer's best friend; aura reading adds uncommon sense, the element in a purchase that otherwise gets lost in the shuffle.

Every purchase is for an individual. Aura reading shows the effects for that individual, here and now.

And you may know less about that individual's reactions than you think. Take shampoo, for instance. Did you ever buy a product that looked great in the magazine but your real-life hair hated it?

Hair stylists recommend that we should switch brands periodically, rather than sticking to one formula forever. But how should you choose that new brand? The packaging, though carefully designed to make you buy, has about as much to do with your actual hair as yummy claims for cat food relate to a real feline's taste. How about buying shampoo from your beauty salon? Should you buy what your hairdresser sells? Or does it make more sense to check prices and brands at the neighborhood drugstore?

New products come out constantly. *Consumer Reports* can't keep up with them all, nor will a top-rated shampoo necessarily suit your particular hair chemistry. People react differently, no matter what the label promises.

That's why, when I crave something new to make me look gorgeous, I drive my aura down to my favorite discount drugstore and test energy. Here's how:

Subtle Shampoo

1. Set an intention to learn about the energy of your hair. Bounce and rub the aura around it. (Choose hair located at the side of your head, avoiding bangs near your third eye, which would be distracting.)

2. With your primary sensor hand ready for an aura rub, ask to feel the energy of your hair now. Feel it.

3. Pick up a product that interests you. This product could be shampoo, conditioner, hairdye, you name it. Check out one product at a time.

4. With your alternate sensor hand, hold the package near your hair. Energetically, this symbolizes using the product.

5. Bounce the aura around your hair. Rub it. Ask about the condition of your hair with use of this product. Compare that information to what you learned in Step #2.

6. Be sure to try several products before you make your choice. For fun, test products you have used recently. You know their physical effects from past experience. It's fascinating to feel the auric equivalent of something you have already tried physically.

   With aura research, I have watched shampoos turn my hair variously lustrous, dull, silky, tangled, bouncy, and overconditioned. Aside from consumerism, this technique is a great way to develop your synesthesia.

7. When you have narrowed down your choices, test any combinations you plan to use together, like Shampoo A plus Conditioner B. More knowledge, more fun!

Question Authority

When it comes to consumerism, you are the ultimate authority, not the salesperson or advertiser. Choose purchases that give you the best value, regardless of how their prices compare. Paying too much isn't desirable. Neither is false economy. Auras can show what a product really does for you.

Here are three of my favorite techniques to distinguish goods from bads.

Aura Test Vitamins

Different manufacturers make products that are more different than you might suppose. As nutritionists will tell you, a vitamin C is not as simple to standardize as the letter C. You probably know about the controversy between organic and synthetic products. But did you know that two competing products, manufactured in the same way, still vary greatly? Find out which brand your body likes best.

1. Next time you go shopping, pick out at least three comparable brands.

2. Hold one bottle to your solar plexus and test your aura.

3. Repeat this for each product you test. See or feel which brand makes the energy bigger, clearer, stronger. You'll be amazed. There really is a difference.

Clothe Yourself With Energy

In the first rapture of falling in love with a garment, you may not notice flaws that could bother you later, like a color that looks less flattering away from the lighting in the dressing room. (Yes, ladies, this is actually possible.) How about a fabric content that will make you itch after five consecutive minutes of wear? Maybe the problem is impossible to perceive physically but still real, like horrible vibes from the sweatshop where the garment was made. Here's your solution.

1. Try on new clothes for beauty, fashion, flatteringness, price—your usual brilliant consumer job.

2. Before you decide to buy any garment, though, try it on differently, for energy. Either read your aura in the dressing room mirror or use your primary sensor hand. Start with an overall view. If you perceive auras in color, make sure the garment doesn't clash!

3. Undress. Take an auric before picture of every chakra whose physical component will be covered by the garment, e.g., for a turtleneck: solar plexus, heart, and throat.

4. Put the clothes on again. Take an auric after picture. If results are satisfactory, you've found clothes worth buying.

Scrutinize Yard Sale Bargains

Triumphs and trophies, that's how my favorite yard sale bargains seem to me when I return from the hunt. It's a great feeling to bring home outrageous bargains you couldn't afford otherwise.

Pay special attention, though, to the energy in personal items: clothing, metal jewelry and precious stones, bedding, towels, shoes. When they touch someone's body repeatedly, they pick up the energy. So you will be buying the past owner's vibes, which may be a mixed blessing. Don't wait until you spot the Al-Anon publications in a box of used books for sale. Test all personal items now.

1. While you're at the yard sale, stake out a corner where you can aura test purchases with relative privacy.

2. Pick up one item at a time. Place your alternate sensor hand on your hip—making a sort of sandwich with the personal item wedged between your hand and your torso. This way you have positioned your potential purchase so you can gauge its effects on your energy.

3. Bend down and use auravision. Otherwise stand up straight and do an aura rub with your primary sensor hand.

4. Pay attention to your root chakra. Maybe you won't feel comfortable in public holding your hand a few inches from your crotch! So rub or look at the energy located around one of the hinges at your thighs, perhaps right next to the hand at your hip.

   This chakra checkup allows you to pay special attention to the effects of purchases on your root chakra. Here's where the most serious energy debris will show up—chronic fear, drug use, physical abuse, traumas. It's a downer to think about such problems but even more of a downer to unwittingly bring them home.

To summarize, **question authority**. That's the slogan every consumer should use along with "In God we trust." Why let advertisers and merchandisers manipulate you into buying? Aside from the personal benefits of spending money wisely, it's your moral responsibility. In the realm of consumerism, every purchase sends an economic message: you vote with your dollars.

Consumers know to look for the facts beyond the hype. I'm not suggesting that aura reading should become your only test of a product. But it can supplement all your other research. And it may turn out to provide your most insightful information.

Materially and metaphysically, both, aura reading enables you to peel off labels and base your evaluation on the situation's true merits.

Hi, Tech

Need help to program your VCR? Sorry, aura reading won't take that problem away. But auras can give you perspective on what today's high-tech gadgets do to your energy field, something well worth knowing.

Now you have the means to assess every gadget in your home and all potential purchases. To test, read your aura. Use the technology. Immediately afterwards, test your aura again.

Question high-tech, especially when it comes to food. Irradiated products are hot consumer items—especially those popular little juice boxes. Manufacturers have demonstrated that irradiation cuts down on spoilage. No harm there, right? But how much life force remains in the package? Find out for yourself before you make it an everyday snack for your kids.

Microwave cooking is another technology aura readers may decide to question. "I never thought I would 'nuke' my food" Kayla told me. "But now that I have kids plus a full-time job, I do it all the time." Those people who don't trust microwaves can easily test their effects on food energy.

As long as you're cooking, why not test the effects of all your kitchen appliances. You need only make the experiment once. Compare fresh food to frozen and canned, organic to commercial. Try baked and broiled, boiled, steamed, slow-cooked, toasted, and raw. It's fascinating.

Recipe for the World's Most Nourishing Food

Here's how to cook up an energy treat for your family: Handle the food directly with clean hands and a loving touch.

Toss that salad without spoons. Mix cookie dough with your fingers. No-tech food, touched by human hands, enriches the ingredients with the cook's consciousness and emotions.

Surrounded by Entertainment

Do your kids question why "sitting too close to a TV isn't good for you"? Teach them to use their hands to feel the energy field six inches from the set. All the technology we use for entertainment has an effect. It's worth considering.

"Surround sound" is an especially pervasive way of taking the entertainment's energy into your aura. What happens with a simple boom box is magnified manyfold with the entertainment centers now being pushed in the stores.

When you're in the store, listen to the salespeople but also listen to your subtle senses. What does your aura feel like after the demonstration? How long does it take for your energy field to bounce back to normal? Research like this may cause you to avoid frequent exposure to huge screens. Or maybe you'll just be selective about what you watch on them.

Sometimes even *unsubtle* perception brings us doubts about technology. You'll see a street kid hooked up to his sound system as if to an umbilical cord. The volume blasts. You want to scream and you wonder if the poor child knows what he's doing to himself energetically.

Given his present state, you'd be a fool ask him. But use auravision or touchy sight to see for yourself.

**Parents, if you teach your own children to perceive
their spiritual energy and value it,
they will grow up paying attention.
Could knowledge like this protect them?**

The point of examining the effects of household technology isn't anti-machine, just pro-human. Some devices, without causing gross physical damage, deaden consciousness. And consciousness is the genuine, natural, home entertainment center.

Think back to your most memorable experiences from books, movies, or videos. The deeper they touched you, the more lasting the impression. Compare that to times when entertainment, sensory overload style, has been entirely forgettable—except for the physical aftermath of exhaustion.

The good news is, some technology really awakens consciousness, presenting profound models of how to use the mind. Telephones, radios, and TVs all have expanded our concepts about how information can travel. It's a prep course for psychic knowing.

Parents laugh about how quickly children master high-tech equipment. Widespread use of computers may be preparing them (and their silly old parents) for future telepathy.

Just learning how to use a word processor can change forever how you conceptualize writing and editing. Electronic gadgets of the future may have the spiritual effect of helping to trigger higher states of consciousness.

Today we have the Internet. It has begun to transform individual users into one giant integrated intelligence. Computers may actually be programming *us*... for enlightenment, a cosmic interconnectedness.

Wedding Presents

The occasion could be a wedding, college graduation, or birthday party. So long as you've got to be present—and probably buy a present—why not get your money's worth: enjoy the energy show.

Every well-planned celebration involves a ritual. Say that William is the guest of honor at the next celebration you're invited to attend. At some time during this event, he will blow out the candle on his cake or receive his diploma, perhaps take a significant spiritual vow.

During rituals, don't just center on facial expressions.
Scrutinize auras.
Great insights may reward you
and sometimes great surprises, too.

For instance, do you cry at weddings? When you watch the auras of bride and groom, you may connect to a wellspring of their emotions, made all the more powerful for being restrained. (Even in these days of casual manners, most fiances restrain themselves. I guess it's common knowledge that engaged persons who sob at the altar may appear somewhat desperate.)

In general, you'll find it fascinating to watch what happens when a person cannot publicly express an emotion that shows strongly in the aura. The impulse to cry or laugh peaks until it leaks—over to the aura belonging to the person most closely connected on a psychic level—that could be the person's spouse or closest friend—or simply the most sensitive empath in the room. As you experienced for yourself in the chapter on "Telephone Awareness," energy dynamics often involve intense give-and-takes.

Often these dynamics include the phenomenon of *psychic ties.* Through this subconscious linkage, one person winds up absorbing and/or expressing another person's emotion. That's why men who never express feelings can have extremely emotional wives, and vice versa.

Also, that's why any time you, the aura reader, start to act out with an intensity that goes far beyond the norm, it behooves you to check the aura of your significant other as well as your own. When you become aware that your spouse or boss or child has a raging power center, that may help you understand why you're screaming. And help you to regain control.

Meanwhile, back at the wedding ... even a secular ceremony with the Justice of the Peace shows its sacredness on an auric level. Watch for this and you'll have one of the most satisfying experiences available to an aura reader. Be especially sure to watch the light show that occurs when the vows are taken.

Shopping for Seminars

"You've just *got* to go," says your best friend. The flyer looks appealing. You can afford to spend the time and the money ... but not if you'll be throwing it away on something with the wrong energy.

Professional seminar givers know that potential customers have their doubts. For that reason, most offer an introductory session before folks sign up for the big package. The importance of attending this session in your role as aura reader cannot be overemphasized.

The topic of the seminar could be God or Amway. Whatever the subject matter, you will be taking an energy bath with this group. The longer the seminar, the larger the group, the stronger the effects.

Frankly, your energy is going to be worked over. That happens when the group is a loving, noncoercive assortment of souls at the perfect vibrational level for you. It also happens in a cult. And until you actually go, you may not know for sure whether the group offers spiritual opportunity, a waste of your time, or danger.

Having worked with many clients who are former cult members, I can assure you that one thing they have in common is the gradual loss of *spiritual self-authority.*

The biblical commandment not to worship idols notwithstanding, it is all too easy to treat a supposed authority like a god on a pedestal. That person becomes the authority about what to believe and what to do. Forgotten is the discipline of seeking truth directly from the still, small voice within.

Eventually self-authority can erode to such an extent that an individual gives away control of his own mind. Individual thinking is replaced with cult thinking: cult langage, cult interpretations, cult self-talk.

When a woman gives her power away to a "movement," she will learn all right, but probably not what she expects. Cults are easy to slip into, hard to recognize. Paradoxically, another common denominator for all cults is that their members never recognize that their particular group is a cult.

Much like addictions to alcohol, drugs, or sex, overdependence on any group eventually ends after a person recognizes that she has gotten stuck and resolves to break free. Once a cult member truly exits, she has learned something vital, never to be forgotten.

Cults. That is the worst case scenario for trying out a new group. Yet even then a person grows. In the best case, a group will gently accelerate your learning, your personal empowerment, your self-authority. And no matter what the nature of your group experience, you will learn faster and smarter when you remember to read auras. The following technique can help.

Group Energy Checkup

This technique will help you assess what is going on aurically with a seminar, organization, or other group. If the group is lovely, you'll enjoy it all the more. And if the group turns out to be a cult, you'll be glad you used this technique to alert yourself.

Even if you are proficient at the technique for reading group body from Chapter Four, use the group energy checkup instead, when you're with strangers. The former technique can bring an experience of spiritual unity, which may not be desirable, depending on the nature of the group. The latter technique brings insight with detachment, more prudent with people you don't yet know.

1. At the start of the meeting, read your aura at the solar plexus chakra for a before picture. Use aura bounce and rub or auravision.

2. During the meeting, have fun watching auras of the regulars in the group and, especially, the leader.

3. Inwardly ask questions to direct your subtle perception. For instance:

- What is the speaker experiencing, spiritually?
  (Look at the speaker's third eye.)
- How does the speaker attempt to involve me?
  (Look at the speaker's solar plexus chakra.)
- Will the speaker tell me the whole truth?
  (Look at the speaker's throat chakra.)
- Is the speaker purposely using sex appeal/charisma
  to keep me involved?
  (Look at the speaker's second chakra.)

4. Jot down notes on your findings, for later questioning with your inner dictionary. For fairness you'll want to interpret what you've discovered, e.g., a charismatic speaker who is truthful and spiritually awake can be wonderful helper, whereas charisma plus dishonesty could be a dangerous combination.

5. Ask your Higher Self to help you spiritually disconnect from the group. This way one is always free to return by choice. However, one will not be drawn back unwittingly, pulled by psychic ties.

6. Immediately after you leave the session, take an after picture of your solar plexus chakra, using the same method as in Step #1.

Use what you learn from this technique in conjunction with your intellectual and emotional reactions to the group and the speaker. Is it for you?

The Search for a Church Home

Who doesn't long to belong? As a person who is spiritually aware, your most important choice as a consumer could be shopping for a spiritual community. A church (i.e., synagogue, temple, mosque, any house of worship) can be valued for many reasons that have nothing to do, strictly speaking, with spirituality. Community confers social advantages, family tradition, and the like. But first and foremost a church is a house of worship.

When you need to find one, aura reading will enable you to do consciously and purposefully what others do vaguely: investigate to what extent a religious service gives a genuine spiritual lift.

The presence of God has been called the still small voice within. It brings a glow that can't be conjured up by philosophizing or emoting. This becomes very clear when you read the aura of the minister, priest, rabbi—whoever is in charge of a religious ceremony.

TV offers convenient opportunities to home shop for religion. Every aura reader should take at least one try at watching the energy of televangelists. These religious leaders are heroes to millions. Beyond their words, what do they communicate?

Turn off the sound. Tune in. Which do you see/feel, a talent for emotionalism or authentic spiritual balance? Does the charisma come from one of the lower chakras? Remembering what you learned in earlier chapters about truthfulness showing in the solar plexus and throat chakras, what's doing? Trust the third eye to reveal the essence of a minister's communication.

Religious theatricals without an inner spirituality are the ultimate separation of church and state (of consciousness).

At the opposite extreme, houses of worship can be stages for genuine performances of spiritual upliftment. Auras of the people in the congregation become larger, clearer, and change in texture. Peek at a worshipper deep in silent prayer or meditation. Now that's a spiritually flashy experience!

During a religious service, aura reading will bring new meaning to old rituals. Does the celebrant just go through the motions or does he move energy?

Traditional rituals become fascinating from this perspective. One friend, a former Trappist monk, told me his perception of the downgrade in energy when the Mass at his neighborhood church changed from Latin to English. "So much of the power was lost." Paul lamented.

"The worst part is that the priest started to face the congregation while preparing the host for communion. He used to face the altar. Energy would come through his crown chakra and out through his back, bathing the whole congregation in light. But when he faced the congregation, the energy bounced off his back and hit the altar instead. The people got a performance. They lost the deeper reason behind it."

That was Paul's vision of things. Someone else might see a different truth entirely, not just because aura readers have different gifts but because of the different intermeshing vibrational levels on this planet. **The bottom line is that you choose the spiritual community to match your vibration.** Aura reading will deepen your understanding of what attracts you spiritually.

Sometimes you may go through a period of time when you cannot find a church home that really suits you. That can be lonely and painful, like being single when you would vastly prefer to be married. But in what kind of a marriage? Avoid joining a church for social companionship when the spiritual part doesn't work. Keep looking. Meanwhile remember this:

With or without a church, you can live with integrity, spiritually awake and striving to grow. Institutions aren't required for you to be kind to others, in service to their highest good.

Even if you have found a church with a spiritual leader who is perfect for you, only you can open your heart to God, which is what spiritual community ultimately means.

When subtle perception develops, you may become more aware of angels—beautiful ones in celestial bodies made of light. Their presence, like God's, is not restricted to churches.

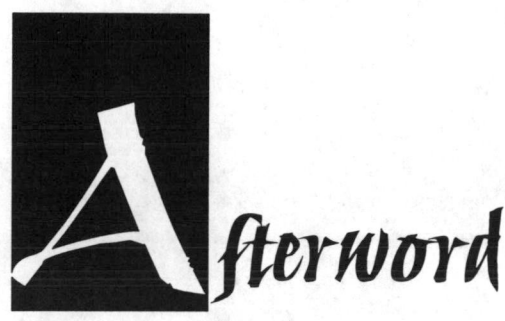

*S*ex was once like auras. For people in my parent's generation, some fifty years ago, public discussion of sex was taboo. Irresistibly, though, people were drawn to consciously acknowledge its importance in everyday life. Here was something private, with a deep and hidden significance, that had fascinating implications for behavior. Folks discussed it with great curiosity but sometimes equally great inhibitions.

My father told me the story of his best friend's secret book. For a month, Irwin carried a certain book with him, reading it whenever he traveled the New York subways. This book generated considerable curiosity because Irwin had made it a cover out of newspaper which he refused to take off.

Adamantly, Irwin refused to answer my parents' questions about what on earth he was reading. As the days stretched into weeks, my father could stand the suspense no longer. When Irwin was out of the room, Dad grabbed the book and opened it up. The title? *Sex without Guilt.*

Maybe you have been similarly secretive about your interest in auras. But actually you are in the forefront of a shift in consciousness. Aura reading is the common knowledge of the future. And by exploring it now, you are helping everyone to wake up to it.

As shown by such scientific phenomena as The Hundredth Monkey Effect, your mind as an individual connects to a group consciousness. When you lift yourself, you lift others. (For more information about this, see Dr. Rupert Sheldrake's book in the Bibliography.)

**On a spiritual level there are no secrets.
As your personal state of consciousness rises,
new information becomes available to you.
As collective consciousness rises, the knowledge from
aura reading will strip many false definitions
and labels from our world.**

Meanwhile, you may seem to be on your own, exploring the secret knowledge of auras. What if your curiosity about auras seems all-consuming? Folks in my father's generation worried (apparently more than young adults do today) about becoming sex fiends. Could you turn into some kind of aura reading maniac?

Such a fear is probably unwarranted. But it is a legitimate concern to keep life in balance. Could you set yourself backwards, spiritually, by reading auras too much? Exactly how much aura reading should you do?

Forget about shoulds. That's my advice.

Discovering auras is a little like falling in love. You fall head over heels, go through a stage where you think about auras constantly, fascinated by how your new perception touches every aspect of your life.

Or aura reading can sneak up on you, the way my husband Mitch sneaked up on me. Before you know what happens, you and aura reading are friends. It adds to your life here and there, unaccountably lifting your spirits. Without much fuss, it becomes part of your life. Eventually, you realize it has become indispensable, a cherished second nature.

So my best advice is to read auras whenever it pleases you, helps you, or helps you to help someone else. Regardless of how often you do these readings, they will demonstrate something important about your level of consciousness.

Give Yourself License

Aura reading shows that you have evolved to a certain level of awareness during your lifetime. Humility and self-doubt notwithstanding, you have a respectably high state of consciousness.

What else did you think you have been doing with all those relationships and romances, those lists of New Year's resolutions, your education—official and otherwise? That goes double if your schooling on Planet Earth has included activities expressly to help you evolve, like psychotherapy, seminars, meditation, contemplation, prayer, saunas, sweats, and good old affirmations.

Every choice you make, every experience has had an effect on you and your aura. Extra! Extra! Now you can read all about it. And every time you read an aura, you *demonstrate* that you have gained a certain amount of spiritual awareness. That's a tribute to all the work you have done so far for personal development.

**A new level of life is opening up to you—
celestial perception—the realm of angels and deep
human secrets. You can look into the heart of things.
Maybe you'll see by looking, maybe you'll feel,
maybe you'll empathically be.**

Periodically you may need to remind yourself to not believe the myth about auras. The test of your abilities is not whether you see cartoon-style bright colors. If you must choose a test, make it joy. How much joy does your reading bring to yourself and others?

Even more than a test, what most of us need is a task. Make it your job to live as an aura reader. Use refined perception to buy a coat, to water a plant. Awareness, like love, is not best displayed by grand promises, but by how you live, day after day.

By reading auras you prove that you have high consciousness. Don't wait for some hypothetical state of enlightenment or a paying client or any recognition whatsoever from anyone to prove that you can know these wonders. You have license because you choose to know. Everyone can.

Perhaps through your example, more people will.

Annotated Bibliography

The scripture and hymns of your religion may be your most important reference books for aura reading. Let them open your heart and lift your vibrations. Add daily spiritual exercises (whatever kinds resonate best for you) and you have the ideal foundation for the method of Aura Reading Through All Your Senses. In addition, the following books may be of special interest.

SPIRITUAL HEALING

At the level of auras and angels, your perceptions will be most reliable when you keep yourself clear of astral debris. The techniques developed by Ann and Peter Meyer for Inner Sensitivity (www.teachingoftheinnerchrist.com. 619-283-4444) can help you to keep yourself clear. Although the techniques are best taught directly through a teacher, Susan Shumsky has done a superb job of making them accessible between covers.

Shumsky, Susan. *Divine Revelation*. New York: Fireside, 1996.

SELF-UNDERSTANDING

Who are you, the aura reader? For starters, you're someone hardwired with learning preferences that last a lifetime. To transcend the Myth about Auras—with its unrealistic expectation that your Celestial Perception must be exclusively visual, even when the rest of your life isn't—explore books about learning styles. They're at least as relevant to adults as to children.

Markova, Dawna Ph.D. and Powell, Anne R. *How Your Child is Smart*. Berkeley: Conari Press, 1992.

Your empathic abilities may intensify when you read auras. Did you know that 1 in 20 people has a significant, trainable gift as an empath? Natural empaths pick up pain that doesn't belong to them. Skilled empaths can turn their gifts on or off at will, including techniques to intensify your clear, direct experience of other people.

Rosetree, Rose. *Empowered by Empathy: 25 Ways to Fly in Spirit.* Sterling: Women's Intuition Worldwide, 2001. www.Rose-Rosetree.com. 703-404-4357.

To learn about empaths and aura readers through fiction:

Rosetree, Rose. *The Roar of the Huntids.* Sterling: Women's Intuition Worldwide, 2001. www.Rose-Rosetree.com. 703-404-4357.

Many of the people drawn to aura reading are introverts. Celebrate your strengths with this compassionate and wise how-to:

Laney, Marti Olsen, Psy.D. *The Introvert Advantage: How to Thrive in an Extrovert World.* New York: Workman Publishing. www.theintrovertadvantage.com. martilaney@sbcglobal.net

Smash boundaries about your perception—and have fun—with all the books in this series:

N.E. Thing Enterprises. *Magic Eye II.* Kansas City: Andrews and McMeel. 1994. www.magiceye.com. 508-487-8484.

PHYSICAL HEALING

Aura reading can help you to become the A+ student of all forms of alternative healing. My favorite book in this field is this immensely practical, accessible and loving how-to:

Eden, Donna. *Energy Medicine.* New York: Jeremy P. Tarcher/Putnam, 1999. www.innersource.net. 800-835-8332.

All the Perelandra publications and products were developed through the clear perception of Machaelle Small Wright. As an aura reader you'll be able to appreciate the superb quality of her work.

Wright, Machaelle Small. *Flower Essences: Reordering Our Understanding and Approach to Illness and Health.* Jeffersonton: Perelandra, Ltd., 1988. www.perelandra-ltd.com. 800-960-8806.

Combine aura reading with a good reference book like the following and you'll gain maximum from do-it-yourself homeopathy:
Cummings, Stephen M.D. and Ullman, Dana M.P.H. *Everybody's Guide to Homeopathic Medicines: Safe and Effective Remedies for You and Your Family.* 3rd ed. New York: Jeremy P. Tarcher, 1997.

SPIRITUAL WISDOM
I'm proud to call this man my mentor. He may have something to teach you, too, about how to balance spiritual awareness with your unique way of being human.
Bauman, Bill Ph.D. *Oneness: Our Heritage, Our Path, Our Destiny.* Arlington: World Peace Institute. 1993. www.billbauman.net.

Aura readers are interconnected, so your daily use of techniques for Celestial Perception can help others. This book will help you to understand why.
Sheldrake, Rupert, Ph.D. *A New Science of Life: The Hypothesis of Morphic Resonance.* Rochester: Inner Traditions, 1995. www.sheldrake.org.

PRAYER
Prayer can be the ultimate volunteer work: Effective, powerful, selfless. Whatever your religious tradition, this Ph.D. in comparative religion can help you to direct your Celestial Perception toward helping others:
Walsh, Birrell, Ph.D. *Praying for Others: Powerful Practices for Healing, Peace, and New Beginnings.* New York: The Crossroad Publishing Company. Birrell leads an online prayer group, too. Find it at http://groups.yahoo.com/group/prayingforothers.

Read your aura before and after doing the techniques in this extraordinary book. Wow!
Blaze, Chrissie and Gary. *Power Prayer.* Avon: Adams Media. 2004. www.chrissieblaze.com. ChrissieBlaze@msn.com.

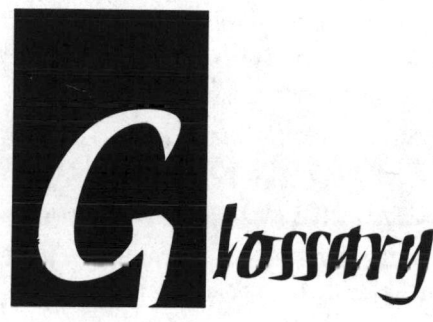

• AFFIRMATION • The verbal declaration of spiritual truth to bring about desired changes in conscious and subconscious thought. Since external reality is an outpicturing of inner conditions, affirmations can improve objective reality along with what is subjective. Effective use of affirmations requires two things: appropriate, powerful *language* to form the structure of the affirmation and *techniques* that engage the mind at the deepest possible level.

• ANALYTICAL AWARENESS • Subtle sense perception through mental agility. For those with this gift, information comes through the mind—including what other people would describe in terms of sight, hearing, touch, and so forth. In addition, the gift of analytical awareness includes unusual facility at moving from level to level of subtle experience, from subtle to subtler.

• AURA BOUNCE • The use of subtle touch for sensing the size and borders of an aura. Since the human aura contains many levels, it is possible to feel more than one energy border. Usually, though, a beginning aura reader will be attracted to one level of aura rather than the others and will gravitate towards that level.

An advanced aura reader can precede the technique of aura bounce with a specific intention to perceive the appropriate level of aura. A helpful way to frame this request is in terms of chakras, since each level of aura corresponds to one of the chakras. Thus, "I wish to touch the level of aura that has to do with the fourth chakra" will reveal this level of aura. It can then be felt all around the body, not only at the position of the fourth chakra.

• AURA READING DICTIONARY • A reference work for personal subtle perception, offering meanings with scientific validity and universal application. Such a dictionary cannot exist because the deepest levels of subtle perception are highly individual.

However, attempts at this dictionary are sometimes published. This happens when an aura reader develops an elaborate system based on personal experience, then offers her dictionary to students as though it had universal validity. While students can train themselves to mimic a teacher's insights, if they push hard enough, their greatest personal contribution as aura readers may come from consulting their own inner dictionary.

• AURA RUB • The use of subtle touch for sensing the quality and content of auric energy.

• AURAS • Energy fields in the form of subtle bodies that wrap around the physical body. Auras are packed with layers of information about what is going on with a person's mind, emotions, health, and spiritual development.

• CELESTIAL CONSCIOUSNESS • An attainable level of spiritual evolution where, at will, one can experience celestial perception. Earth is a learning planet where the path to higher consciousness includes mastery of the subtle senses, synesthesia, and the choice to seek spiritual development. The purpose of this book is to give readers the techniques that will bring them to celestial consciousness. However, no book can substitute for the guidance of a personal teacher.

• CELESTIAL PERCEPTION • Direct personal experience of deeper levels within physical reality. Celestial perception is located at the level of the seed form (*see* Glossary definition). Beauty, delicacy, and joy are typical attributes of celestial perception.

• CHAKRA • Energy center within the aura. Each person has seven main chakras (as well as the numerous secondary chakras not covered in this book), and each chakra is responsible for an area of functioning of the mind-body-spirit system.

• CLAIRAUDIENCE • The subtle sense of hearing. This perception shows itself through appreciation of nuances of sound, resonance, and silence. Information also can come through inner hearing of words.

• CLAIRSENTIENCE • The subtle sense of touch. Clairsentient perception can come through touching the physical body or the aura.

• CLAIRVOYANCE • The subtle sense of sight. Clairvoyance can involve a variety of perceptions, such as light (colored or not), patterns of energy, even knowledge that comes as a result of looking but involves no visual flash at all.

• DENIAL • Being consciously unaware of the truth, avoiding unpleasantness. Sometimes considered a necessary defense mechanism, denial doesn't make serious problems go away and, in fact, can make them worse. Health problems, for example, often involve denial. Patterns of chronic denial can show in the energy field. Aura readers may learn to detect them, even help heal them.

• EMOTIONAL EMPATHY • Taking on the emotional state of another person as though it were one's own. A trained empath uses this form of subtle perception by staying aware of "personal" feelings and questioning their origin.

• EMOTIONAL TOUCH • Relating to auras through awareness of emotions. Information reveals people's underlying feeling states.

• ENLIGHTENMENT • A spiritual goal of life, where a person knows the truth of reality to an extent that liberates the soul from pain, fear, confusion, and unnecessary limitation. When enlightened, one's sense of identity is based on being an energy presence, rather than a name, a job, a nationality, etc.

• EXPECTATION • A psychological or spiritual obstacle to spontaneous experience. Often a person can consciously substitute intention *(see* Glossary definition*)* for expectation. It's the difference between letting a desire be known to Spirit and dictating the precise manner of the desire's manifestation.

• EXTRASENSORY PERCEPTION • (E.S.P.) Information from any of the 11 faculties of subtle perception identified in this book. Commonly this "extra" sensing is not acknowledged in everyday life because it goes by quickly and is not consciously understood. Learning about the subtle senses and training them through the techniques in this book can make a great difference in using these inborn gifts.

• GROUNDING BREATH • Out-breaths that puff the air out hard enough to make a blowing sound paired with shallow in-breaths through the mouth and nose together. Combined with the intent to connect with the physical environment, grounding breaths bring awareness back to physical reality.

• GUSTATORY GIFTEDNESS • The subtle sense that involves smell or taste. Sometimes it brings information in the context of healing. Always it links awareness to other subtle senses. The highly individual symbolism of subtle taste and smell is explained by the inner dictionary.

• HIGHER SELF • Language for referring to one's inner spiritual source. Depending on one's belief system one could, alternatively, call this God, a spiritual master such as Jesus or Buddha, the angels, one's Higher Power, or one's inner wisdom.

• HOLDING A SPACE • The ability to pay attention to people in a deeply receptive way. A common example of this gentle, unfocused awareness is known as "bonding" between a baby and the primary caregiver. For an aura reader to consciously become aware of holding a space, and do this often as part of aura reading, can strengthen the subtle senses of holistic knowing, emotional empathy, and physical empathy.

The ability to link to others in consciousness, when trained, can be especially useful for telepathy, prayer, and leadership on the level of group body. Note: Space can be held for any intelligent being, including plants and animals.

• HOLISTIC KNOWING • Subtle sense perception through making connections. For a person with this gift, clearest aura reading occurs when seeking information that relates people, ideas, and resources. Holistic awareness involves holding a space big enough for a variety of things to harmonize perfectly, however briefly.

• INNER DICTIONARY • A set of information written in consciousness deep within the individual. Consulting this dictionary enables a person to interpret subtle perception in a way that is productive as well as meaningful. Each person's dictionary is unique, flowing out of subjective perception and connected to the spiritual work only that person can do.

• INTENTION • The basis for some of the most powerful techniques that involve consciousness, will, or intelligence. Setting an intention requires three steps: putting in a specific request to one's Higher Self (*see* Glossary definition); open-ended expectancy of good (i.e., trust that the request will be granted in the best way possible); letting go.

• KINESTHETIC • Using the subtle sense of touch. *See* Clairsentience.

• PHYSICAL EMPATHY • Taking on the physical sensations of another person as though they were one's own. A trained empath uses this form of subtle perception by staying aware of "personal" bodily sensations and questioning their origin.

• PSYCHIC KNOWING • The subtle sense that works like truth knowledge, physical empathy, and emotional empathy all rolled into one—and available long distance. This includes experiencing the auras of people far away in time and space. Interestingly, the quality of this experience may feel very personal, not remote at all.

• SEED FORM • The subtlest, most causative, of all layers of creation. It is the spiritual equivalent of DNA. Aura readers have the potential to experience a range of subtlety about every physical object in creation. To "read the seed" requires the most profound inner quiet and physical calmness. From this level of experience, an aura reader can connect with knowledge about any of the subtle senses.

• SELF-AUTHORITY • Making oneself the ultimate human decision maker about what constitutes personal spiritual truth.

• SENSES • Languages to convey the spiritual reality of life. From a metaphysical standpoint, each material object has a seed value. This essential vibration translates simultaneously into the language of the physical senses. This book identifies clairaudience, clairsentience, clairvoyance, emotional touch, and gustatory giftedness as the five subtle versions of the physical senses.

These, plus the "sixth senses" discussed in this book, are ways to explore physical reality in pursuit of spiritual knowledge.

• SENSOR POSITION • Useful hand position for subtle perception. To do: Cup your hands, as if you were about to hold water in them. Separate hands, still keeping fingers and thumbs close to the palm of each hand. Each of these "energy mitts" can be used independently to touch and experience the aura.

By contrast, when a hand is not in sensor position, fingers spread apart. Energy leaks through the fingers. Therefore, sensor position makes more energy available for subtle touch. This intensifies the clarity of kinesthetic perception.

• SEX • Commonly sex is understood to involve pleasure, release of sexual tension, procreation, and emotional intensity. For an aura reader, sex has additional significance. Sexual arousal and intercourse are ways to turn up the level of energy in the mind-body-spirit system.

Whether alone or partnered, sexual release can balance, expand, and cleanse the chakras. There are tremendous advantages, however, to sexual partnership. Assuming that both partners begin with all chakras open, they have the opportunity to merge all parts of the energy system regardless of whether physical orgasm takes place.

• SIXTH SENSE(S) • Subtle faculties of knowing. They are an invaluable asset for aura reading. This book identifies six: emotional empathy, physical empathy, analytical awareness, holistic knowing, psychic knowing, and truth knowledge.

• SOUL TRAVEL • A shift in consciousness where your primary sense of who and where you are moves from your physical identity to another person or place. This experience is far easier and more common than most people are aware; though soul travel happens *in consciousness*, it may not *be conscious*. Aura reading techniques, such as The Heart of the Heart, can facilitate intentional experiences of soul travel.

• SYNESTHESIA • The senses working together, the deep inner connection of all 11 subtle senses. People are often tempted to use mixed metaphors to describe their deepest experiences. One reason is the desire to communicate with images and symbols that combine many senses, rather than sorting information into single-sense, specialized categories. The method of Aura Reading Through All Your Senses involves the intentional use of synesthesia to enliven all subtle senses.

• TELEPATHY • The spiritual ability to merge consciousness with another intelligence. This sharing brings knowledge that can be used in practical ways. However, as a spiritual experience, the degree of clarity for the perceiver is inversely proportional to the amount of ego involvement. Unlike "mind reading," telepathy has no connotation of trespass into the consciousness of another for personal gain.

• TRUTH KNOWLEDGE • The subtle sense version of knowing. In practice, it means a person doesn't know how she knows, she simply knows. Truth knowledge is triggered by subtle hearing, smelling, touching, and so forth that bypasses the perceiver's conscious recognition.

• UNWELCOME PERCEPTION • Experiences and information about subtle reality that the aura reader finds undesirable. Learning to read auras should include learning what do about unwelcome perception.

• VIBE-RAISING BREATHS • Long deep in-breaths through the nose and out-breaths through the mouth. The in-breaths can connect conscious awareness with the Higher Self. The out-breaths help to release negative emotions and stress. Combined with the intent to advance spiritually, this breathing pattern shifts one's spiritual energy to a higher frequency.

• WAY IN • Each individual's process of opening to clear and meaningful subtle perception. Finding one's way in is like discovering and pushing a button that opens the door to a secret passageway.

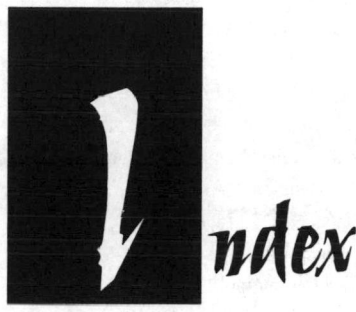

For a complete listing of every technique in this book, see the Table of Techniques.
Bolded numbers show the most important reference for each topic.

For a complete listing of every technique in this book, see the Table of Techniques.

For a complete listing of every technique in this book, see the Table of Techniques.

For a complete listing of every technique in this book, see the Table of Techniques.

For a complete listing of every technique in this book, see the Table of Techniques.

S

For a complete listing of every technique in this book, see the Table of Techniques.

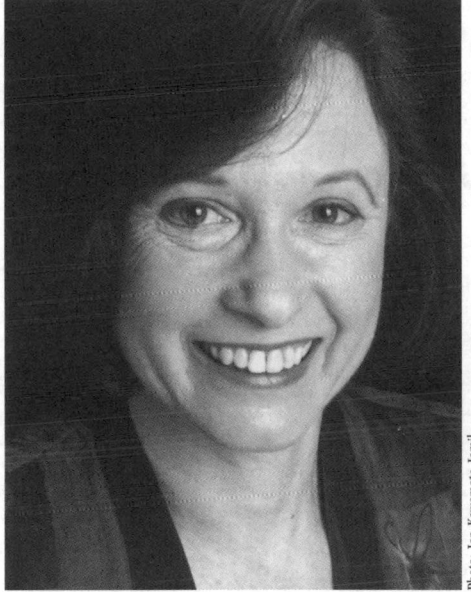

Photo: Jan Kawamoto Jamil

Rose Rosetree

Since 1971, Rose has taught techniques to develop Celestial Perception in everyday life. Currently she offers workshops in her specialties of face reading, aura reading, body language and training for skilled empaths. Personal sessions for spiritual awakening and emotional healing are also available.

For details about all these resources, plus free articles about the auras and faces of people in the news, click on www.Rose-Rosetree.com. Within the U.S., sessions and books can be ordered at 800-345-6665.

Media interviews for this award-winning teacher have brought Rose's insights to Europe, Asia, Africa and Australia. In America, interviews include ABC's "The View," *USA Today, The Washington Post, The Washington Times, The L.A. Times, Ladies Home Journal, Redbook* and "The Diane Rehm Show."

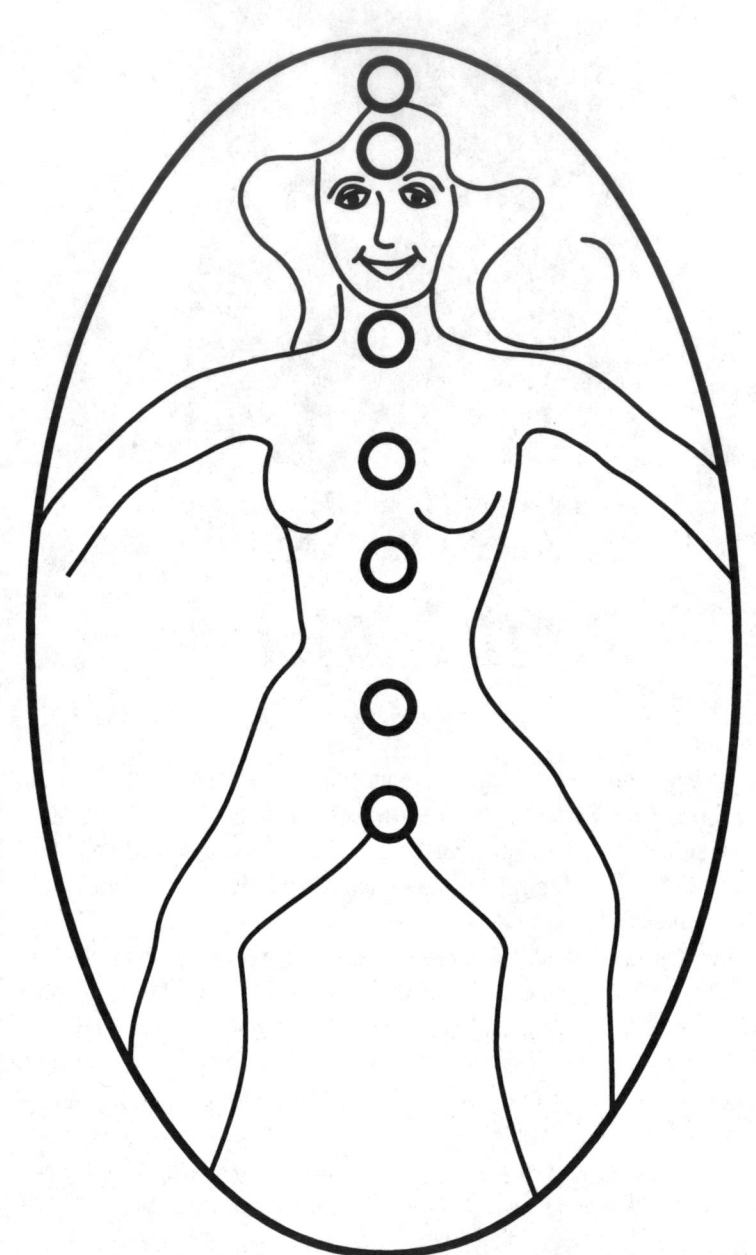

The Seven Main Chakras as Information Centers

Chakra	Gives Information About
1. Root	Trust vs. mistrust
2. Lower Abdominal	Sexual energy, childlike creativity, psychic awareness
3. Solar Plexus	Power vs. victimization
4. Heart	Giving love and receiving love
5. Throat	Freedom of self-expression
6. Third Eye	Spirituality, willingness to look at life
7. Crown	Receiving spiritual energy

Read People Deeper

It's easy to order these life-changing books. Within the U.S., call 800-345-6665. For secure ordering online (including international orders) click on **www.Rose-Rosetree.com.**

- **Aura Reading Through All Your Senses** $14.95

- **50 Ways to Read Your Lover:** $14.95
  Compatibility Revealed in Body Language,
  Face Reading, Auras & Chakras

- **The Power of Face Reading** $18.95

- **Wrinkles Are God's Makeup** $19.95

- **Empowered by Empathy** $18.95

- **The Roar of the Huntids (Novel)** $22.95

- **Thrill Your Soul (Video)** $24.95

Note: Prices listed here subject to change without notice.

Also Available Now

Rose's monthly zine (Internet magazine) gives you face readings and aura readings of people in the news. It's fun and it's free. To subscribe, send an email with the message SUBSCRIBE to Rosetree@Starpower.net.

You can work directly with America's leading expert at deeper perception. Choose from face readings, aura readings and personal sessions. (Fees start at just $15.) Details at www.rose-rosetree.com or send a stamped self-addressed envelope to WIW, 116 Hillsdale Dr., Sterling, VA 20164.